Self-Assessment Co[...]

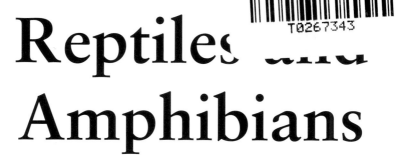

Reptiles and
Amphibians

Second Edition

Frederic L Frye
BSc, DVM, MSc, CBiol, FSB(FIBiol), FRSM
Diplomate (Honorary) American Board of Veterinary Practitioners
(Reptile/Amphibian)

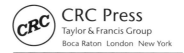

CRC Press
Taylor & Francis Group
Boca Raton London New York

CRC Press is an imprint of the
Taylor & Francis Group, an **informa** business

CRC Press
Taylor & Francis Group
6000 Broken Sound Parkway NW, Suite 300
Boca Raton, FL 33487-2742

© 2016 by Taylor & Francis Group, LLC
CRC Press is an imprint of Taylor & Francis Group, an Informa business

No claim to original U.S. Government works

Printed and bound in India by Replika Press Pvt. Ltd.

Printed on acid-free paper
Version Date: 20150623

International Standard Book Number-13: 978-1-4822-5760-1 (Paperback)

Visit the Taylor & Francis Web site at
http://www.taylorandfrancis.com

and the CRC Press Web site at
http://www.crcpress.com

Dedication

To Brucye, Lorraine, Erik, Noah and Ian. To Dr. Wilbur Amand, Executive Director of the Association of Reptile and Amphibian Veterinarians (ARAV), who so skillfully and generously shepherded that organization since its inception; and to my colleagues and dear friends, Professor Giovanni DiGuardo, who exemplifies the very best in professional collegialism, and Dr. Douglas R. Mader, who has achieved every potential that I recognized in him when he was a student of mine in the 1980s.

Acknowledgements

I want to express my appreciation to my colleague, Dr. Douglas R. Mader, for reviewing and making numerous insightful comments on the manuscript for this book. The following colleagues generously contributed case material and/or photographic or radiographic images:

Case number	Contributor	Case number	Contributor
4	Mr. Clifford Warwick	163	Dr. Christopher Katz
31	Dr. Angelo Lambiris	173	Dr. John Allan
40	Dr. Pavel Siroky	174	Dr. Robert Altman
87	Dr. Nicasio Brotons	175	Dr. Caroline Pond
98	Dr. Pavel Siroky	177	Dr. Walter Rosskopf
99	Dr. Zahi Aizenberg	180	Dr. David Huff
116	Ms. Erika Sorenson	182	Mrs. Jeri Hegenbart
118	Dr. Nathan Cohen	183	Dr. Ana Salbany
119	Dr. Fabio Faiola	184	Dr. Christopher Katz
132	Dr. Alvin Atlas	191	Dr. Howard Schwartz
134	Mr. Brian Gray	192	Dr. Betsy Rodger
136a-e	Dr. Oscar Grazioli	201	Dr. Marta Avanzi
136f	Dr. Stephen Goldberg	204	Dr. Andi Milhaca
		213	Dr. Angelo Lambiris
153	Dr. James Corcoran	220	Dr. Bogdan Cordos
156	Dr. Chris Knott	221	Dr. Allejandro A. Bayon del Rio
157	Dr. Bogdon Serpy		
158	Mr. Clifford Warrick	224	Dr. Andi Milhaca
159	Mr. Clifford Warrick	226	Dr. Rachel Blackmer
160	Dr. David Huff		

Broad classification of cases

Alimentary system: 3, 10, 22, 26, 48, 103, 105, 119, 153, 165, 176, 180, 199, 220, 223

Anatomy (normal structures): 54, 67, 81, 85, 115, 117, 128, 129, 148, 193, 194, 195

Anesthesia: 161

Dermal/integumentary conditions: 4, 12, 27, 36, 53, 74, 79, 87, 98, 122, 133, 137, 141, 147, 149, 150, 185, 197, 214

Developmental anomalies: 25, 35, 52, 114, 130, 132, 134, 177, 178, 213

Endocrine disease: 72, 175

Environmental conditions: 15, 36, 100, 112, 118, 158, 207

Foreign bodies: 15, 48, 106, 162, 176, 187

Hematology: 2, 16, 29, 32, 37, 41, 62, 84, 86, 95, 107, 109, 142, 145, 190, 209, 215

Identification of animals: 31, 43, 59, 61, 65, 76, 111, 120, 123, 124, 127, 152, 168, 184, 196

Infections: 5, 24, 70, 74, 91, 99, 101, 102, 104, 105, 108, 113, 131, 137, 138, 139, 140, 142, 144, 147, 150, 153, 155, 156, 157, 164, 167, 169, 179, 218, 220, 223, 232

Neoplasia: 39, 40, 98, 172, 173, 181, 191

Neurological dysfunction: 104, 151, 153, 205, 232

Nutrition/nutritional disorders: 3, 10, 13, 14, 20, 23, 50, 56, 69, 71, 93, 97, 106, 116, 126, 149, 166, 180, 208, 227, 229

Ophthalmic disorders: 11, 15, 79, 159, 202, 208, 211, 212, 219, 221

Parasites: 9, 18, 24, 34, 38, 39, 42, 44, 45, 49, 55, 58, 60, 63, 66, 73, 77, 78, 87, 92, 110, 121, 171, 203, 204, 206, 210, 212, 216, 217, 224

Renal disorders/excretion: 1, 7, 30, 64, 88, 96, 113, 125, 126, 172, 228

Reproductive system: 19, 47, 68, 75, 80, 81, 82, 83, 85, 89, 94, 100, 115, 124, 125, 129, 136, 143, 163, 173, 177, 178, 182, 188, 198, 207, 226

Respiratory disease: 70, 139, 141, 162, 174, 225, 231

Skeletal system: 21, 33, 39, 57, 91, 99, 135, 140, 160, 169, 186, 201, 218, 230

Trauma: 11, 17, 46, 51, 75, 183, 189, 192, 200

Contents

About the author

Fredric L. Frye
BSc, DVM, MSc, CBiol, FSB (FIBiol), FRSM, Hon. Dipl. ABVP (R/A)
After his honorable discharge from the US Navy, where he served as a combat air crew member in a blimp squadron engaged in antisubmarine patrols, Fredric Frye earned his degrees at the University of California, Davis and served two residencies: General Surgery with an emphasis on cardiovascular surgery at the US Public Service Hospital, San Francisco, and Pathology at the University of California, Davis. He is an elected member of two scholastic honor societies: Alpha Gamma Sigma and Phi Zeta. He was an epidemiologist with the California Cancer Research Program and then engaged in private clinical practice in Berkeley and Davis, California. Dr. Frye joined the faculties of the University of California School of Medicine, San Francisco, teaching experimental surgery; University of California, Berkeley's Lawrence Berkeley Laboratory, working on nuclear medicine, immunosuppression and space-suit design for the NASA Apollo Project; and the University of California, Davis, School of Veterinary Medicine, as a Clinical Professor of Medicine serving pro bono for 24 years. In 1977 he returned to the University of California, Davis, and earned a Master's degree in Comparative Pathology. For 23 years, he was the principal pathologist for a biopharmaceutical research firm until they relocated to the United Kingdom in 2005. He is now a Visiting Professor of Comparative Medicine and Pathobiology at numerous Universities and Colleges in North America, UK, Italy and Japan. He is the author of 23 textbooks, four non-scientific books, 363 papers, 38 CD Rom programs; and co-author of 28 textbooks and numerous chapters in multiauthored textbooks. He has authored three humor titles, *Phyllis, Phallus, Genghis Cohen – and Other Creatures I Have Known*; *Politicians and Diapers Should Be Changed Frequently – and for the Same Reason*; and *May I Inquire as to What the Chicken Did*. His memoir, *Pa Ba La Ba La Gum*, was published in 2014.

He was the 1969 recipient of the American Veterinary Medical Association's Practitioner Research Award; he was the second Edward Elkan Memorial Lecturer at the University of Kent, the Richard N. Smith Memorial Lecturer at the University of Bristol, and the Peter Wilson Bequest Memorial Lecturer at the University of Edinburgh. He is an elected Life Member of the American Association for the Advancement of Science and an Elected Fellow of the Royal Society of Medicine and the Institute of Biology, London. He was named as a Patron of the Charles Louis Davis Foundation for International Advancement of Veterinary and Comparative Pathology and was elected to the Board of Directors of the German Society for the Study of Comparative Pathology and Oncology in Berlin. In 2001 he was elected as an Honorary Life Member of the British Veterinary Zoological Society.

After developing – and maintaining – an intense interest in animals in general, and particularly reptiles, amphibians and invertebrates, he applied his clinical veterinary skills to these previously overlooked animals and has been credited by his colleagues as the 'Father of Herpetological Medicine and Surgery'. In January 2002, he was honored as the recipient of the first Association of Reptilian and Amphibian Veterinarians (ARAV) Lifetime Achievement Award, which now is named the Fredric L. Frye Lifetime Achievement Award. In 2010, he was named as the first Distinguished Honorary member of the Associazione Linnaeus in Italy. The multiauthored text, *Invertebrate Medicine*, to which he contributed a chapter on scorpions, received the 2012 TEXTY AWARD. In 2013 he was awarded a Lifetime Membership in the ARAV, and in 2014, Fred was honored with an Honorary Diplomacy in Reptiles and Amphibians by the American Board of Veterinary Practice for his contributions to Herpetological Medicine and Surgery.

Retired from private practice, Fredric consults on difficult clinical cases with colleagues; mentors students; and devotes much of his time to the family certified organic farm, *La Primavera*, where he is engaged in pomological culture and improvement of apple, pear, peach, plum, nectarine and citrus fruit trees. In the 1980s he was successful in producing viable garlic seeds from a plant that usually reproduces only asexually. Among his avocations are designing and building fine furniture and sculpting art objects from sustainable tropical forest products, metal and stone; he has had two one-man shows of his artwork.

Preface

The first edition of this book was written with a retrospective view and deep appreciation of comparative medicine, surgery and comparative pathology in its broadest sense. As the author of this second edition, permit me to give my assessment of where I perceive herpetological medicine and surgery has come and where I think it will continue to progress into the future.

'One Health' was a concept emanating from joint meetings of officials of the American Medical Association and the American Veterinary Medical Association. It was a notion that was long in coming and is a most welcome advance in thought. After all, humans are animals. We share many of the same maladies. Physicians deal with but one species and two genders, while veterinarians deal with anywhere from two to several thousands of species (depending upon one's specialty), and as many as six genders (male, female, ovariectomized females and castrated males, intersex individuals, and even uniparental parthenogenetic animals). Beyond those differences, however, both professions approach their patients in much an identical fashion, and strive to achieve the same goals employing the same diagnostic and treatment techniques. These approaches certainly apply to the so-called 'lower' vertebrates as well as to human and non-human mammals.

Radiography, in all of its highly useful expressions including plain and contrast imaging, ultrasonography, magnetic resonance and three-dimensional computed tomographic scanning, nuclear isotope tracing, and so forth, is used for producing images as diagnostic tools. Physiological chemistry for analyzing blood, urine and other bodily fluids, and routine histological processing and, where indicated, highly specific immunohistochemical staining, are essential diagnostic laboratory techniques that aid in the precise characterization of neoplastic and other abnormal tissues. Doppler blood-flow detection and echocardiology are advances in diagnostic medicine that find ready applications in herpetological medicine and surgery. Often, the main obstacles to the application of some of these diagnostic modalities are access and cost. That stipulated, numerous academic and private practices now offer those diagnostic modalities. The advent of new and highly effective anesthetic agents, antibiotics, anti-inflammatory agents, and non-steroidal analgesic medications has brought the practice of herpetological medicine and surgery into the mainstream of veterinary medicine and surgery. When I graduated from veterinary school 50 years ago, many of these technologies and chemical agents were not available because they had not been invented! Commencing in the 1960s, a more realistic approach began to evolve, and as it did organized herpetological medicine and surgery became a reality. There were, however, sceptics who thought that treating reptiles and amphibians was a waste of their precious time and efforts. Those opinions did not prevail, and herpetological medicine and surgery eventually became a veterinary discipline that warranted formal recognition and board status – both of which it has justifiably earned.

Much has happened in the 19 years since the first edition of this book was published. Many more scientists and clinicians have taken an interest in reptiles and amphibians. As a result, the membership in the Association of Reptile and

Amphibian Veterinarians (ARAV) has grown exponentially, and more veterinary schools and colleges are now including academic coverage of the care and treatment of these non-domestic animals in their curricula. Crucially, in the years since the first edition was released, many individual species of amphibians, especially frogs, have become extinct, owing in part to habitat loss and, increasingly, the highly contagious fungal organism *Batrachochytium dendrobatidis*, which continues to devastate populations in Australia and South, Central, and North America. In late 2014, a second species of this mycotic pathogen, *Batrachochytium salamandrivorans*, was reported from European urodele amphibians.[1] This species of *Batrachochytium* was imported with salamanders originating from Southeast Asia, some of which may represent a novel source of healthy carriers of this organism. Unfortunately, this pathogenic fungal taxon has already been isolated from tailed amphibians in The Netherlands and Belgium. Because of its inherent pathogenicity for many species of urodeles as well as populations of amphibians native to continents where native newts and salamanders lack natural immunity, this new newly discovered chytrid poses a threat to amphibians far from its point of origin. Cryptosporidiosis, because of a parasitic protozoan pathogen, is ever more frequently diagnosed in captive reptiles and, like several viral diseases of reptiles, is a major concern of captive collections and breeders. Numerous bone diseases, some of which are linked to nutritional deficiencies/excesses, and captive environmental husbandry are common in reptiles and amphibians. The precise laboratory determination of normal physiological values and the application of these analytical investigations to actual cases of infectious, nutritional, metabolic, parasitic, and neoplastic diseases are of significant importance to the early diagnosis and effective monitoring of numerous treatment regimens.

During the past two decades many novel radiographic techniques have been developed and are now placed at the disposal of veterinary clinicians, especially those attached to academic institutions and, as noted previously, also in some private practices. Clever veterinary surgeons have devised operative solutions to numerous serious conditions in both reptiles and amphibians.

Thus, for these reasons and the enthusiastic acceptance of the first edition, the publishers decided that the time was right for an expanded second edition. The choice of whether to include cases and images from the first edition was left to my judgment. I wanted to keep this edition fresh and of interest to my colleagues who have the first edition on their bookshelves – and in their memories. In addition, I kept in mind the value of many of those cases for training younger generations of veterinarians and students. In the first edition, and in this one, the reader is presented with the facts of the cases and may be asked to give a diagnosis, treatment or management plan, prognosis, or a rational means for preventing a certain condition; or to identify a particular parasitic organism, what measures to take in instances of multiple cases within a collection or colony situation, and so forth. As was the case with the first edition, the cases are purposely presented in a random fashion because in actual clinical practice, that is exactly how cases occur. Unless a clinician is a specialist, she or he is unlikely to see multiple or consecutive cases of a dermatological or ophthalmological condition in a series of one after another;

nor is one likely to have an endless number of metabolic or infectious disease cases without other diagnostic challenges comprising radiological, diagnostic laboratory investigative, or surgical procedures mixed in between the others. Also, there are instances where the reader is questioned as to the identification of a particular animal, blood cell, parasitic ovum or cyst. This form of presentation is also a means for sustaining interest in pursuing the self-assessment format. Also, in the 'real' world, one does not have the luxury of filling out a college blue book when faced with a clinical challenge. Rather, one must think, consider the facts revealed in the history, the signs shown by the patient, the laboratory results, and so forth, and winnow through several possibilities, then formulate a rational answer that includes likely diagnoses, a cogent treatment plan, and prognosis.

There is a bias in the selection of cases inasmuch as certain species of reptiles and amphibians are more often kept as 'pets' or study animals. Thus, there are more boa constrictors, green iguanas, Old World chameleons, certain monitor lizards, African frogs and toads, American alligators, North American and European turtles and tortoises and some other tropical and temperate-zone snakes than might be expected. These are the taxa that are more often sold by pet dealers and, consequently, are more likely to be seen by veterinarians.

Pioneers of comparative medicine such as the 17th century's Marcello Malpighi, the 18th century's John Hunter and the 19th century's Rudolph Virchow contributed mightily to our fund of knowledge via their experimental approaches, which included non-mammalian species. Each was a physician-pathologist, and they all shared an intense interest in investigating, in an integrated manner, the intimate anatomical and physiological relationships of cells, organs and entire organisms. Rather than merely investigating a sole entity, a solitary lesion, or an isolated organ or organ system, each explored insights that evolved into an integrated – dare I say – 'holistic' approach to a given patient. Individually those cells, organs or organ systems are interdependent (i.e. each and every part of an organism exerts an influence on its counterparts). The herpetological patient, be it a frog, toad, newt, salamander, snake, lizard, tortoise, crocodile or any other creature, must be seen and appreciated as the whole of its disparate parts.

From this, one can see that obtaining a thorough history is absolutely essential. Not only the details of the individual patient, but also:

- What environmental factors might have played a role in inducing a particular condition or disease to appear?
- How many animals in the collection are unwell or have died?
- Has microbiological and/or toxicological testing been carried out?
- Have histological examinations occurred?
- Is a quarantine program established and if so, for how long and how is it managed?
- Was nutrition per se or some deficiency in a major or minor nutritive component a contributing factor?
- What is the source of the dietary items fed?
- Did a traumatic event occur?
- Was a mixed population of animals housed together?

- Was hyper- or hypothermia involved as a contributing factor?
- What is or was the age of the patient(s) when the disorder was first manifested or noticed?
- Did other animals in the immediate environment of a particular patient also exhibit signs of a similar disease or disorder?
- Have there been recent additions to the animal colony?
- What protocols or measures are in place for cage or colony hygiene?
- What, if any, treatment has been administered to this and/or any other animals in the collection?
- What is the nature of water management?
- What is the source of drinking water?
- Is the water treated, and if so, how and with what agents or equipment?
- How is that treatment delivered or applied?
- What cleaning or sanitizing products have been used, and how often and by whom?
- Have there been changes in the personnel responsible for the care of the animals?

These are but a few of the epidemiological questions that must be asked and answered in order to assess fully whether there is any commonality in a disease outbreak in a collection or colony of captive animals. It may seem lengthy or bothersome to some observers, but these questions are essential in order to fully investigate deaths, especially in instances of multiple losses.

Obviously, the economic considerations of any particular situation play a role. The fees charged by a diagnostic laboratory for analyzing blood, urine, tissue, food, water, and so forth are often as much as or more than those fees charged for humans or conventional domestic animals. That fact being stipulated, the economic value of many captive reptiles and amphibians often justifies expensive laboratory investigations – particularly if the animal is a cherished pet or a very expensive exotic species, when multiple animals are involved in a disease outbreak and/or when the disease is communicable to humans. In some instances, legal and/or forensic issues remain to be considered and resolved, and, again, these justify the expense of professional expertise.

Long gone are the days of inexpensive, 'disposable' imported animals destined for the 'pet' trade. Import regulations are strict and the wholesale trade of highly restricted or forbidden CITES-identified species is now under close scrutiny; legal convictions now carry much stiffer sentences of monetary fines and imprisonment. Because of these factors, the forensic investigation of criminal cases involving captive reptiles and amphibians has become more commonplace in North America, Europe, and Asia.

In addition, veterinarians, especially comparative pathologists, may be called upon to serve as expert trial witnesses and give sworn testimony in cases involving reptiles and amphibians. Be forewarned, the courts demand precision in all means of documentation and testimony; the defense will surely pounce on any perceived lapse in either of these essentially important components!

In some instances, the identification of a particular species is requested. I have asked this question only in certain instances when that identification was vitally important. For instance, when an animal is toxic or venomous to humans, or when a species is CITES-listed and should not be in private hands unless legally permitted and accompanied by appropriate documentation.

For many decades, I have counseled qualified veterinarians and veterinary students to perform complete necropsies on all patients who are encountered dead on arrival, or who die on the operating table or whilst in the care of a veterinary clinician. It is astonishing what can be learned from these necropsies and how often one's initial impression or tentative diagnosis is incorrect. This type of instruction is absolutely invaluable – and essential – for acquiring expertise as an accurate diagnostician, thus making for a much better clinician when dealing with living patients!

This edition also differs slightly from the first in that although the majority of the images shown are from my own clinical archive, many others are from esteemed colleagues who have kindly and very generously shared their clinical cases and pertinent details and images. Their contributions are cited, giving credit for photographs and/or case materials.

I hope that you, the reader, will enjoy this excursion into self-assessment.

Fredric L. Frye

[1]Martel, A, *et al.* (2014). Recent Introduction of a chytrid fungus endangers Western palearctic salamanders. Science 346(6209):630–1.

Abbreviations

AST	aspartate transaminase
CNS	central nervous system
CPK	creatine phosphokinase
CT	computed tomography
DIC	disseminated intravascular coagulation
EDTA	ethylenediamine tetra-acetate
H&E	hematoxylin and eosin
HPOA	hypertrophic pulmonary osteoarthropathy
IM	intramuscular
IV	intravenous
MRI	magnetic resonance imaging
NSHP	nutritional secondary hyperparathyroidism
PAS	periodic acid–Schiff
PCR	polymerase chain reaction
PCV	packed cell volume
RBC	red blood cell
SC	subcutaneous
SCUD	septisemic cutaneous ulcerative disease
SGOT	serum glutamic oxaloacetic transaminase
UV	ultraviolet
WBC	white blood cell

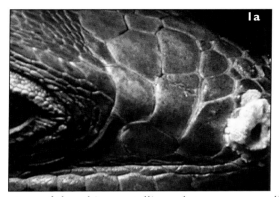

1i. What is the nature of the white crystalline substance surrounding the external nares of this female Central American iguana (1a)?
ii. What is its significance?

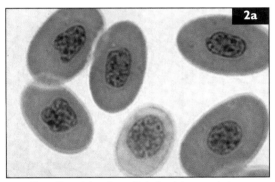

2i. Identify the small cell with the slightly blue-staining cytoplasm amongst the larger erythrocytes in the following thin blood film, stained with benzidine peroxidase from a snake (2a).
ii. What is its primary function?

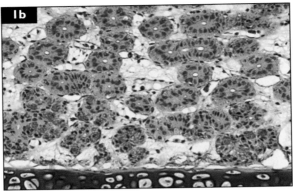

1i. The crystals are salt, NaCl and lesser amounts of KCl.

ii. Some terrestrial and marine reptiles utilize non-renal excretion of some electrolytes in order to help maintain osmolar equilibrium without losing significant volume of essential water. This excretion is accomplished by nasal salt glands that are located beneath the nasal mucosa. (See **1b**: Histological section of nasal salt glands from a green iguana.)

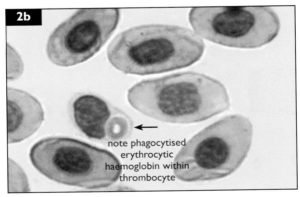

note phagocytised erythrocytic haemoglobin within thrombocyte

2i. A thrombocyte.

ii. Its primary function is blood coagulation. It can also function as a phagocyte when called upon during bacterial infection and/or during excessive erythrocyte destruction (**2b**)

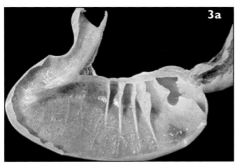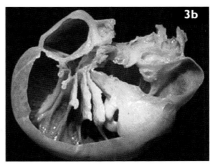

3 The following two images illustrate a portion of the alimentary system of two green iguanas, a juvenile (**3a**) and an adult (**3b**).
i. What is the anatomical term for this organ?
ii. What is the function and significance of this organ with respect to the nutrition of these lizards?
iii. What organism is critically important in this metabolic processing of complex plant carbohydrates into useful nutritional constituents?

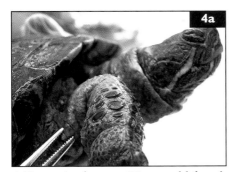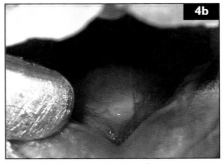

4 Figure **4a** shows a 25-year-old female red-eared slider turtle, *Trachemys scripta elegans*, with a grossly thickened integument and firm pale plaques on the lingual tip. Figure **4b** depicts lingual tip lesions on the tongue of the same turtle.
i. What is your interpretation of this turtle's condition?

3 i. These are the sacculated colons from an immature iguana and a mature adult. The wall has been excised to show the interior lumen whose surface area is expanded by the presence of extensions into the lumen. Note the difference in appearance between the juvenile and adult organs. It is in these multiple sub-chambers that fermentation occurs and reflects the dietary change between the two age populations.

ii. These organs serve as hind-gut fermentation sites where plant materials undergo fermentation. Complex carbohydrates, such as cellulose, are degraded into simple sugars and fatty acids, especially propionic acid, analogous to what occurs in the multichambered fore-stomachs of ruminants.

iii. The principal protozoon responsible for carbohydrate fermentation within the sacculated colon is *Nyctotherus* sp.

4 i. Scleroderma. This is an autoimmune disease most often, but not invariably, affecting (female) humans. Two representative photomicrographs of this interesting relatively rare disease in the turtle are shown below (**4c, d**). Note the epidermal hyperkeratosis and mineralization of the dermis.

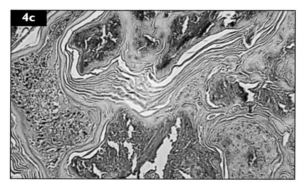

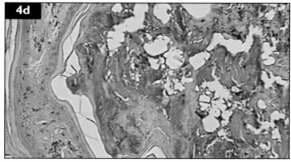

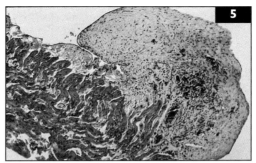

5 Figure 5 is a stained histological section made from the myocardium and endocardium of a boa constrictor (*Boa c. constrictor*).
i. What is your interpretation?
ii. How would you diagnose this condition antemortem?
iii. How would you treat a patient with a similar lesion?
iv. What is your prognosis for an animal with an identical lesion?

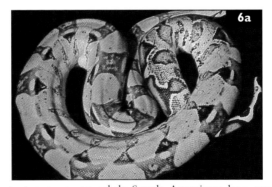

6 Figure 6a illustrates a young adult South American boa constrictor (*Boa c. constrictor*) with multifocal palpable firm swellings and an inability to straighten out from a curled position. The snake was otherwise bright and alert and would eat if presented with freshly killed rodent prey. The signs occurred very gradually over a period of at least 1 year.
i. What are some provisional diagnoses?
ii. How would you investigate this patient's disorder in order to formulate a diagnosis?
iii. What is the treatment, if any, of this condition?
iv. What is your prognosis?

5 i. The confirmed diagnosis was chronic granulomatous vegetative endocarditis.

ii. A lesion such as this one can be diagnosed antemortem via (1) Doppler blood-flow detection and/or (2) ultrasonographic scanning/echocardiography.

iii. Treatment, after appropriate microbiological culture and antibiotic sensitivity testing, would consist of intensive specific antibiotic administration, anti-coagulant treatment to help prevent infective thrombophlebitis and thrombo embolism and careful and compassionate nursing.

iv. The prognosis is guarded to grave. Dissemination of detached fragments of infective thrombi are commonly associated with these lesions.

6 i. Provisional diagnoses include multiple vertebral traumatic or pathological fractures, multifocal osteomyelitis, osseous neoplasia, multifocal vertebral osteofibrosis and osteitis deformans (Paget's disease of bone). The confirmed diagnosis in this and numerous other similar cases was osteitis deformans. (See Figures 6b–e.)

ii. Diagnostic investigations include plain-film radiography, ultrasonography, CT or MRI scanning, image-assisted core-needle biopsy and histopathology.

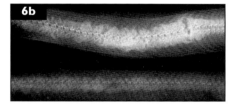

6b

iii. There is no treatment shown to be effective.

iv. The prognosis is guarded to grave.

6b Plain radiograph of boa constrictor's spinal lesions. Note that the ribs are largely spared from the exuberant bony proliferation.

6c Cleared osteological specimen of affected boa's vertebral column. Note that the ribs are minimally involved in the proliferative process.

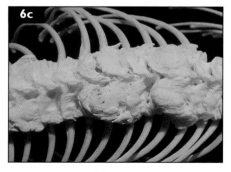

6c

6d Stained thin histological section of affected decalcified vertebral bone. Note the characteristic mosaic pattern created by the irregular cement lines.

6e Micrograph of normal reptilian bone shown for comparison.

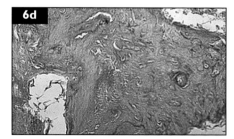

6d

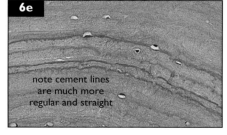

6e

note cement lines are much more regular and straight

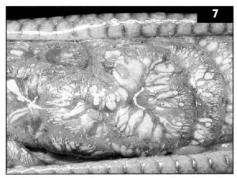

7 Figure 7 was recorded during the necropsy of a North American rat snake (*Elaphe* sp.), and is focused upon one of the kidneys; the opposite kidney was identical to this one.

i. What is your diagnosis?

ii. What are some of the major etiologies for the induction of this condition?

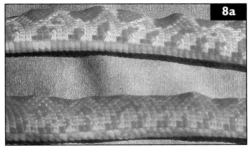

8 Figure 8a shows the appearance of two sibling red color hypomelanistic-morph North American corn snakes (*Elaphe guttata*). Both snakes developed multiple firm swellings that involved their vertebral columns before they were 1 year old.

i. What are some tentative provisional diagnoses?

ii. What tests or diagnostic procedures would you use to assist in determining the true nature of these lesions?

iii. What are some etiological possibilities?

iv. What advice would you offer to the owner of these snakes?

7 i. Visceral (renal) gout. This is the accumulation of urate crystals in the renal tissues causing obstruction of urine processing and flow through the collecting system of the renal system.

ii. Etiologies for visceral gout include:

• Water deprivation.

• Acquired renal damage and/or scarring from infection involving the glomerular and ductal collecting system.

• Any of several toxic agents that affect the kidney tissues. These include bacterial and mycotin renal infections and several nephrotoxic drugs such as aminoglycoside antibiotics. Also, inadequate attention to supplemental fluid intake to maintain renal perfusion while on antibiotic therapy; some industrial chemicals; numerous toxic plants; renal neoplasms; and some protozoon and metazoon parasitic organisms.

• Any extramural or extrarenal obstruction that diminishes urine flow through the kidneys.

8 i. Tentative diagnoses include multifocal traumatic fractures, multifocal osteomyelitis, bony and/or cartilaginous neoplasms, familial fibrous dysplasia. The histopathologically confirmed diagnosis was fibrous dysplasia.

ii. Diagnostic tests include radiological scanning and fine-needle biopsy.

iii. Etiological possibilities are multiple traumatic or pathological fractures, pathological bacterial, fungal, protozoon or metazoan parasitic organisms inducing multifocal sites of osteomyelitis, benign or malignant neoplasms.

iv. Because of the identical lesions occurring in siblings, the possibility or likelihood that the etiology of these masses share a common, probably genetic or epigenetic etiology, the parents should not be rebred and all of the offspring from this clutch of eggs should not be distributed to other collections or breeders.

8b Histological section of one of the lesions. Note the fibrous invasion and displacement of the cancellous spaces that would normally be filled with bone marrow cellular elements.

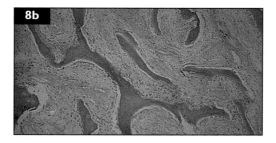

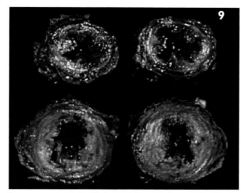

9 Figure 9 shows four sections of the colon of a mature South American boa constrictor (*Boa c. constrictor*). The colonic mucosa is grossly thickened and inflamed.
i. What is the protozoan organism often associated with inducing this form of colonic inflammation?
ii. What other major organ is often severely involved with infection by this organism?
iii. What is the standard treatment for this infection?

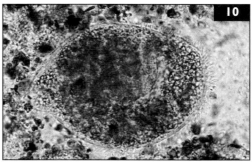

10 Figure 10 is a photomicrograph of a merthiolate-stained organism from the feces of a green iguana (*Iguana iguana*); very similar organisms are found in Australasian bearded dragon lizards.
i. Identify the organism.
ii. What, if any, is the treatment for ridding the host of this organism?
iii. Why?

9 i. *Entamoeba invadens*.

ii. The liver is often also involved in this form of amebiasis.

iii. The treatment for this protozoan parasitism is metronidazole 20–40 mg/kg (depending upon the species of reptile being treated) repeated in 14 days.

10 i. The organism is *Nyctotherus* sp.

ii. This ciliated protozoon is **essential** for nutrition, in that it is a principal fermenter of complex carbohydrates, converting them into simple sugars and long-chain fatty acids.

iii. This organism is not a parasite, but rather, a commensal. Thus a lizard in which this organism is identified does not warrant treatment. In the event that a lizard has been treated with metronidazole (or other amoebacide) that has killed the normal gut flora, the sterilized gut can be repopulated by feeding fresh feces from a healthy, non-parasitized lizard.

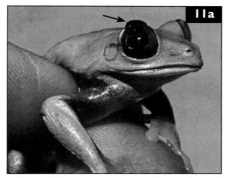

11 Figure **11a** is of a Central American red-eyed tree frog (*Agalychnis callidryas*) with a prolapsed iris protruding from its right globe. The history of this case revealed that the frog was kept with others of its species in a terrarium whose interior was furnished with plastic artificial plants and misted every few hours with freshly collected rain water; thrice weekly live crickets were placed in the terrarium.
i. With the above history, what is a likely etiology for the iris prolapse?
ii. What measures could be implemented to prevent a recurrence of this condition?

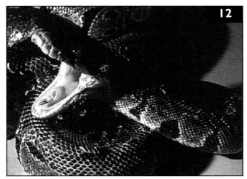

12 Figure **12** shows a ball of regal python (*Python regius*) with multiple integumentary abnormalities.
i. How do you interpret this snake's condition?
ii. What is the most likely etiology?
iii. What visceral organ is likely to be affected?
iv. How would you treat this snake?
v. What recommendations would you make to the owner of this snake to prevent a recurrence of this condition?

11 i. This is an example of cricket-bite trauma (11b).

ii. This trauma could have been avoided if a suitable food for the crickets had been provided to them. Fresh leafy vegetables should always be in terraria and cages as fodder for living crickets.

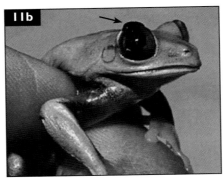

12 i. This snake appears to be suffering from dysecdysis and, quite likely, severe dehydration. It's senescent epidermis has failed to shed properly during at least one, and probably other, ecdyses. The open-mouth breathing can be attributed to retained epidermis obstructing the external nares and/or dessicated mucus within the respiratory tract.

ii. Most snakes imbibe water from vessels that contain suitable volumes and/or depths that permit them to partially immerse their mouth.

iii. Following severe subacute or chronic dehydration, the kidneys are often affected by hyperuricemia and visceral gout.

iv. The snake should be rehydrated with appropriate physiological fluid via *parenteral* adminstration. The snake should also be soaked for at least a half-hour in slightly tepid water, then its now-softened retained epidermal fragments gently removed with a moistened towel. If necessary a few drops of contact wetting solution can be added to the retained spectacle(s) and/or in greater volume bath water to aid in softening the fragments.

v. The owner should be informed of the necessity to have a container of fresh water available in cages at all times.

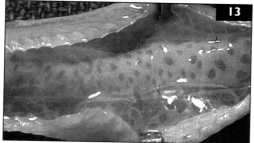

13 Figure 13 illustrates the interior body wall of a snake during a necropsy examination.

i. What is your interpretation or diagnosis?

ii. What is the etiology?

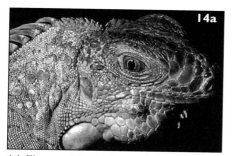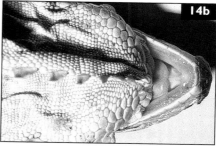

14 Figures 14a, 14b are lateral and ventro-dorsal views, respectively, of a long-term captive adult green iguana (*Iguana iguana*) affected by signficant mandibular shortening.

i. This shortening is characteristic of what common nutritional disorder?

ii. Why are the mandibles so much more affected than the bones of the skull?

iii. Can you suggest a course of treatment for this lizard?

iv. What is the prognosis?

v. Can anything be done to remodel and lengthen the mandibles?

13 i. The multifocal red lesions are charactreristic of serous atrophy of fat.
ii. The etiology is chronic starvation/inanition.

14 i. The manidibular foreshortening is one of the characteristic features of nutritional secondary hyperparathyroidism. The mandibles, like other bones in the affected lizard's skeleton, become softened. The tongue is attached just inside the center of the lower jaw and also to the sternum. The result is that the tongue tends to exert traction on the softened mandibles and causes them to withdraw caudally and bow outward.
ii. The skull bones are usually equally osteoporotic, and, thus, softened; however, because they do not have retractive muscular forces acting upon them, they do not display as much distortion.
iii. Treatment is directed toward improving the diet so that the calcium:phosphorus ratio of the foods fed are at least 2:1. Extra calcium in the form of calcium gluconate, calcium carbonate, etc. and supplementary oral vitamin D-3 are also advised. Calcitonin salmon has also been used to great effect. It lessens the osteolytic activity of osteoclasts, while not adversely affecting osteoblastic activity. Whenever possible, exposure to natural or artificial UV radiation with the appropriate wavelength should be provided to aid in the synthesis of natural vitamin D-3.
iv. The prognosis is favorable with respect to remineralizing the osteoporotic bones. However, the mandibles usually do not return to their previous length, because they are under retractive forces from the lingual musculature
v. The mandibular rami can, with larger iguanas and other lizard patients, be surgically lengthened by one or more bilateral wedge osteotomies. Fine orthopedic wires are utilized to support the wedges of bone while they are reversed and inserted to elongate and unite the mandible. It is delicate orthopedic surgery and most

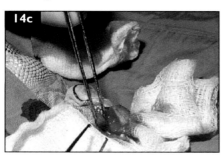

owners usually decide not to pursue it for economic reasons. Figures **14c–e** are intraoperative photographs and a radiograph of the procedure applied to this same iguana. At the conclusion of the surgery, the mandibles were successfully lenghtend to near, but not quite, normal length.

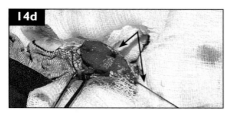

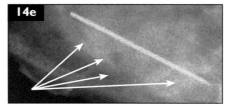

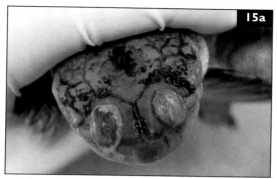

15 This African side-necked turtle, *Chelodina expansa*, was presented with bilateral severely inflamed conjunctival and integumentary tissues (**15a**). It had been maintained in an aquarium filled with fresh water, aquatic plants and abundant algae.

i. What tests or procedures would you employ to ascertain the nature of the severe bilateral inflammation?

ii. How would you treat this patient?

iii. What is your prognosis?

iv. What can be done to lessen the chance of recurrence in the future?

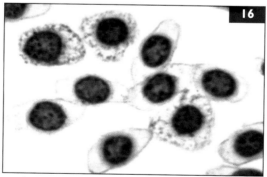

16 Identify the erythrocytic cells characterized by their basophilic stippling in this new methylene blue-stained blood film from a European Hermann's tortoise (*Testudo hermanni*) (**16**).

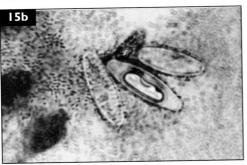

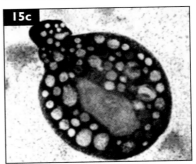

15 i. Cytological and microbioloigcal culture and sensitivity examination of exudates are indicated.
ii. Thorough but gentle lavaging of the affected tissues with physiological saline and topical application of a soothing ophthalmic ointment pending laboratory results. Figures **15b**, **15c** show photomicrographs of the cytology of stained exudate. Note the macrophage filled with diatomaceous debris. Note the myriad number of bacteria and the four diatoms. These organisms are characterized by their silicon cell walls. This glass-like material is exceedingly irritating to delicate tissues such as those surrounding the eyes. Once the diatoms were identifed, an antibiotic ophthalmic ointment containing corticosteroids was applied three times daily. Within 1 week the inflammation had subsided. After another few days, the turtle opened its eyes and began to feed.
iii. The prognosis is favorable once the offending foreign bodies have been removed and the inflammation has resolved.
iv. Frequent water changes and removal of exuberant algal growth should reduce the likelihood of recurrence.

16 They are reticulocytes, juvenile erythrocytes.

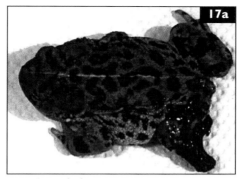

17 A female Western toad (*Bufo boreas*) (17a) was injured by a falling object and sustained a crushed left hind-limb. From the examination, the injury had occurred at least several days prior to the toad being presented for evaluation.

i. How would you manage this severely traumatized patient?

ii. Considering that the toad's injury was to one its its hind-limbs, what is the prognosis for this animal being able to survive after being released to its native habitat following recovery?

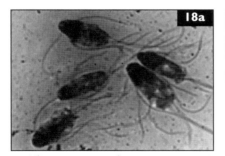
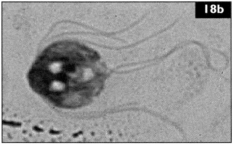

18 The organisms shown (Figures 18a, 18b) were representative of approximately 60 others recovered from the turbid fluid aspirated from the coelomic cavity of a female Pacific pond turtle (*Actremys marmorata*).

i. Identify these organisms.

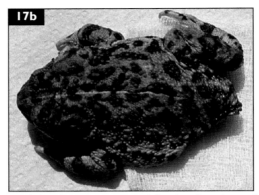

17 i. The toad was stabilized with parenteral fluids administered via intracoelomic infusion, broad-spectrum antibiotics by intramuscular injection, and its injured limb gently but thoroughly cleansed and debrided. During debridement, it was clear that total amputation was indicated. Once it was stabilized, the toad was anesthetized and a coxo-femoral disarticulation amputation was performed.

ii. The prognosis is favorable. Upon recovering from anesthesia, the toad made several attempts to hop but, as expected, it went in circles. However, in less than 1 week, it had learned to crawl, rather than hop and was able to catch its insect prey without difficulty. The toad was rephotographed approximately 2 weeks after having its hind-limb amputated and it was released. Seven months later, it was observed doing very well in the author's garden. An immediate postoperative image of the toad is shown (**17b**).

18 i. The flagellated organisms are *Hexamita* sp.

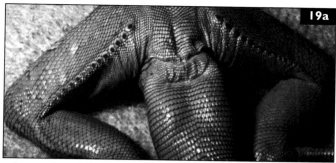

19 What is the gender of the green iguana illustrated in Figure **19a**?

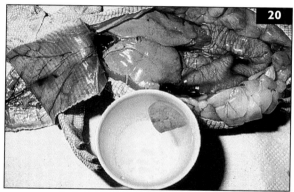

20 Figure **20** was recorded during necropsy examination of an adult savannah monitor lizard (*Varanus exenthematicus*). Note the color of the liver and the piece of liver floating in a cup of water.
i. Why is the liver tissue so bouyant?
ii. What is the most common etiology of this condition?
iii. What measures can you take to prevent this condition?

19 It is a male. Note the paired hemipenial bulges and prominent femoral pores aligned on the ventral surface of each hind-limb (**19b**).

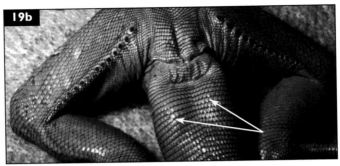

20 i. The liver is bouyant because it contains an abnormal amount of intracellular fat. The proper term for this condition is hepatic steatosis (hepatocellular lipidosis).
ii. Although several other etiological factors *can* induce this condition, the most common one is chronic obesity from overfeeding.
iii. The most effective measure to take in order to prevent this disorder is to feed these captive-housed lizards less to avoid obesity. Under natural (wild) conditions, these lizards forage almost daily, but only occasionally secure a prey meal. Doing so requires them to exercise. Remaining in a cage where they rarely expend much energy and being fed too often leads to gross obesity, which can induce other metabolic disorders.

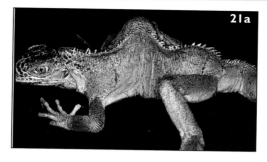

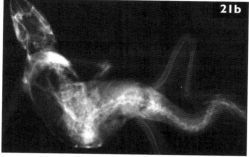

21 i. What is the medical term for the condition shown in Figures 21a, 21b of a green iguana (*Iguana iguana*)?
ii. What is the etiology for this condition?
iii. In a breeding colony situation, what advice would you offer?

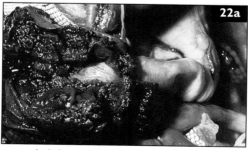

22 Figure 22a was recorded during the necropsy of a mature green iguana (*Iguana iguana*).
i. What is your diagnosis, based solely upon this solitary photograph?
ii. What are some etiologies for this condition?

21

21 i. The medical term is kyphoscoliosis.
ii. There is a strong genetic component with respect to its etiology.
iii. Because of its heritability, affected individuals and their parents should not be selected as breeders.

22 i. Intussusception of the ilium into the saculated colon.
ii. Two common etiologies are:
* Severe infestation with intestinal helminths, especially pinworms, *Oxyuris* sp.
* Severe chronic inflammatory bowel disease.

Figure **22b** is a stained thin histological section of another lizard's intussuscepted intestines, illustrating how one section of gut has telescoped into an adjacent loop. The black pigmented serosal surfaces of the each segment are readily identified and is a common feature of some diurnal lizards.

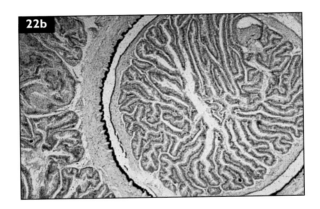

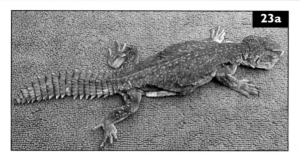

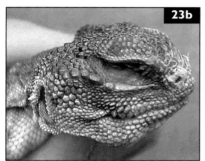

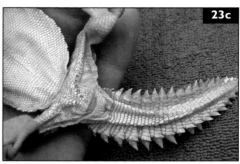

23 Figures **23a–c** are views of a male African uromastyx lizard (*Uromastyx* sp.).
i. What is your interpretation of this lizard's physical condtion?
ii. How would you treat this patient?
iii. What is your prognosis?

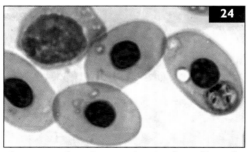

24 Identify the two intracytoplasmic parasites in the cell on the far right of Figure
24 of erythrocytes from a chelonian.

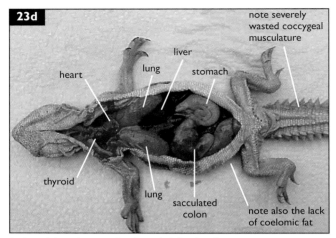

23d note severely wasted coccygeal musculature
liver
heart
lung
stomach
thyroid
lung
sacculated colon
note also the lack of coelomic fat

23 i. Chronic inanition (starvation) and dehydration.
ii. This lizard should be handled gently whilst it is rehydrated with parenteral physiological fluids and tube fed via gastric gavage with readily digested and assimilated nutrient preparations. Alimentation should be of only high-quality, but *modest* protein content early in treatment to protect the kidneys (see Figure **23d**).
iii. The prognosis is guarded, particularly because of the profound dehydration, which may already have induced hyperuricemia and visceral gout-related renal shut-down. This lizard has little, if any, reserves upon which to call, if further stressed.

The lizard died and Figure **23d** was recorded during the necropsy. Note specifically the severe muscle wasting, lack of intracoelomic fat and microhepatica (shrunken liver).

24 The large blue object at the lower end of the cell is *Plasmodium* sp., and the clear, 'signet' object to the left of the erythrocyte's nucleus is *Chelonoplasma* sp.

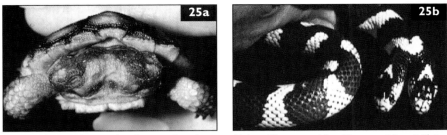

25 i. What is the medical term for the condition illustrated by Figures **25a, 25b**?
ii. Can such animals survive in the wild?

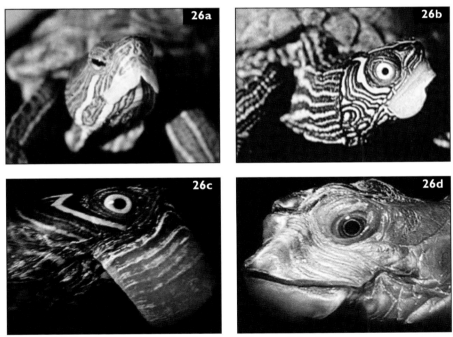

26 The four semi-aquatic turtles shown in Figures **26a–d** share a common lesion involving their tomia (keratinized mouthparts).
i. What is the etiology for this condition?
ii. How would you manage these cases?
iii. What measures can you recommend to prevent this condition from recurring?

25 i. Bicephaly.
ii. Yes. Numerous examples of adult two-headed reptiles have been recorded. The California king snake (*Lampropeltis getulus californiae*) shown was captured as an adult. The neonate desert tortoise, however, would be highly unlikely to survive either in the wild or as a captive because its heads are so far apart that it would probably not be able to eat by itself.

26 i. This condtion of tomial overgrowth occurs in captive animals, rather than wild chelonians, and is induced by the absence of abrasive sufaces on which these animals rub their mouthparts while feeding. Also, it can be related to the lack of abrasive food sources such as snail shells, etc. that are normally present in a more natural diet.
ii. These overgrown mouthparts are easily trimmed with a rotary saw, burr file or sanding disk.
iii. Adding bricks, large stones, pieces of scabrous coral and small snails or empty snail shells to the aquatic environment will afford ample opportunities for turtles to abrade their mouthparts. If a sanding disk or rotary file is employed to trim and reshape the overgrown keratinized tissues, care must be exercised to avoid overheating the remaining healthy tissues.

27 i. What is the condition affecting this South American boa constrictor's (*Boa c. constrictor*) right eye (27a)?
ii. How would you manage this patient's problem?

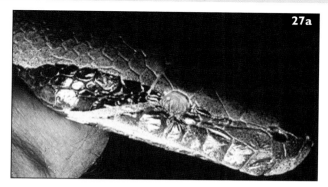

28 i. Identify the intraethrocytic organisms shown in Figure 28 of stained whole blood from a diamondback rattlesnake (*Crotalus atrox*).
ii. What is their clinical significance?

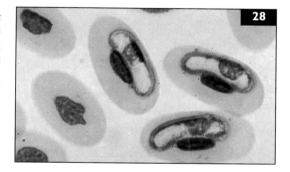

29 Figure 29 is of a stained blood film from a semi-aquatic turtle.
i. Identify the two non-erythrocytic cells.

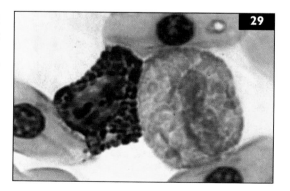

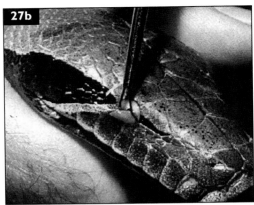

27 i. The boa shown has retained the senescent tertiary spectacle that is normally detached and lost each time the snake sheds its epidermis during ecdysis.

ii. The safest means for detaching retained spectacles is to first moisturize the site with ophthalmic wetting solution until the tissue softens, and then using a cerumin loop, to gently lift the spectacle from the underlying new one covering the cornea (**27b**).

28 i. Hemogregarines (*Hemogregarina* sp.).

ii. These organisms are clinically insignificant, except that they are usually only identified in wild-caught reptiles. Thus their presence can be used as a forensic indicator as to whether an affected reptile probably was *not* captive-bred.

29 i. A basophil (left); a heterophil (right).

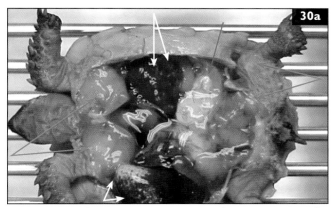

30 The necropsy image shown in Figure **30a** is of an immature African spurred tortoise (*Geochelone sulcata*) that died after approximately 3 years in captivity. Specifically look at the visceral and periarticular tissues (colored arrows).
i. What is your diagnosis?
ii. What are some major etiologies of this induced condition?

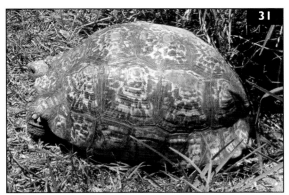

31 Identify the animal illustrated in Figure **31**.

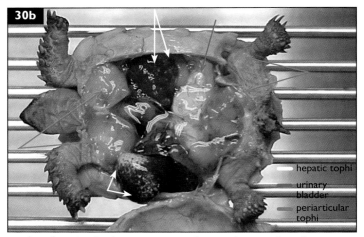

30b
hepatic tophi
urinary
bladder
periarticular
tophi

30 i. Visceral and periarticular gout, secondary to hyperuricemia.
ii. Major etiologies for acquired hyperuricemia and gout are:
• Water deprivation, dehydration.
• A protein-rich diet not suited for a herbivore.
• Renal insufficiency related to acquired kidney disease, including infections, parasitism, neoplasia, etc.
• Extrarenal urinary flow obstruction.
• The ingestion of some nephrotoxic chemicals; the administration of some antibiotics, especially aminoglycosides.
• The ingestion of some nephrotoxic plants.

Figure **30b** is color-coded showing: black, hepatic gouty tophi; red, urate-filled urinary bladder; pale green, periarticular gouty tophi.

31 An adult African leopard tortoise, *Geochelone pardalis*.

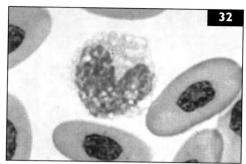

32 Identify the blood cell in the center of Figure 32.

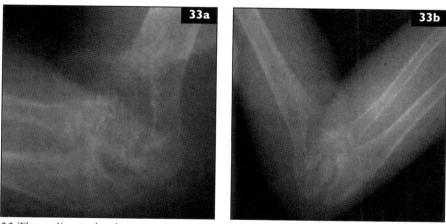

33 The radiographs shown in Figures 33a, 33b were made of the limbs of an adult female iguana (*Iguana iguana*) that was presented for severe and chronic lameness. Both radial-humeral and both femoral-tibial joints were involved; only the fore-limb lesions are shown.
i. What is your diagnosis?
ii. What is the etiology?
iii. How would you treat this patient?
iv. What is the prognosis?

32 A monocyte. Note the deeply indented nucleus and pale blue-staining cytoplasm with numerous clear vacuoles.

33 i. Chronic rheumatoid arthritis.
ii. It is known to be an autoimmune disease in humans and is likely to be in this instance also.
iii. Treatment consists of analgesics (for example meloxacam at a dosage of 0.05–0.1 mg/kg SC or orally) to control pain and corticosteroid administration to diminish inflammation of the synovial and other periarticular tissues.
iv. The prognosis is guarded because the articular and periarticular tissue damage is already extensive.

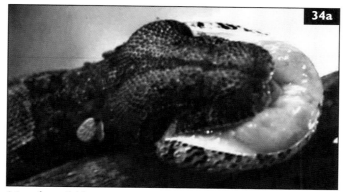

34 Figure **34a** of a wild boa constrictor (*Boa constrictor imperator*) was recorded in a Central American rain forest.
i. What is your diagnosis of this snake's condition?
ii. What are likely etiologies that induced this condition?
iii. How would you treat this snake?
iv. What is your prognosis?

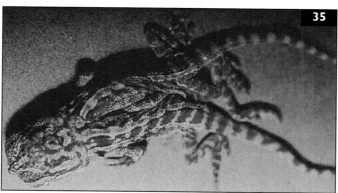

35 How would you describe the anatomical condition illustrated in Figure 35?

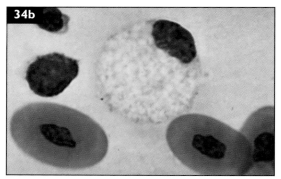

34 i. Acute allergic reaction; severe acute angioneurotic edema.
ii. This response is usually induced by a histaminic reaction to an allergen. Note the two mating ticks attached to the snake's upper cervical region and others on its skin. It is possible that the snake is reacting to a foreign proteinaceous substance originating from the ticks.
iii. Treat the snake with an injectable antihistamine such as diphenhydramine HCl and, if necessary, a rapid-acting corticosteroid. Remove the ticks.
iv. The prognosis for recovery is favorable. Interestingly, blood films made from this snake prior to treatment reveal marked degranulation of eosinophilic leukocytes (34b).

35 Axial, postcephalic duplication. This form of duplication is much less common than bicephaly.

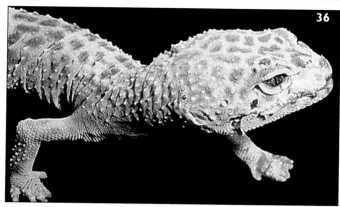

36 i. What is your interpretation of the leopard gecko (*Eublepharis macularius*) shown in Figure 36?
ii. What is its etiology?
iii. How can it be prevented?

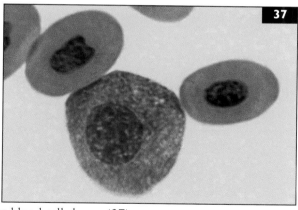

37 Identify the blood cell shown (37).

36 i. Dysecdysis-related autoamputation of several digits.

ii. Ringlets of retained partially shed old epidermis, when moistened and then dry, can shrink and function as mini tourniquets, thus obstructing blood flow to tissues that are distal to the constriction. Often these geckos will actively grasp and ingest shards of partially shed skin. Importantly, these geckos' natural habitats are usually relatively humid. However, when they are maintained in a very dry terrarium habitat, these lizards, often suffer from dysecdysis related to an overly dry cage environment.

iii. This condition can be prevented by increasing the cage relative humidity to approximately 50–60%.

37 An azurophil. Note the nearly spherical nucleus and azurophilic finely granular cytoplasmic inclusions or stippling.

38 Figure **38a** is a metazoan parasite. Match the image with the ova in Figures 38b–e.

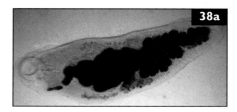

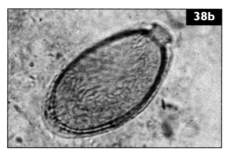

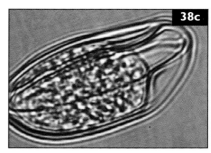

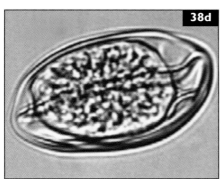

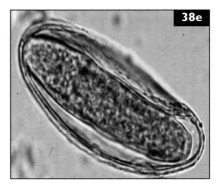

39 i. What is your interpretation of the radiograph in Figure **39** of an Australasian bearded dragon (*Pogona vitticeps*) lizard's left fore-limb?
ii. How would you confirm your diagnosis?
iii. How would you treat this patient?

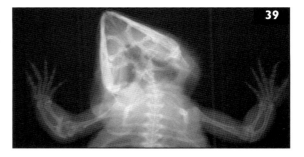

38 The organism shown is a trematode (fluke); the correct ovum that matches the adult is 'b' a trematode ovum. Note the single operculum at one end.

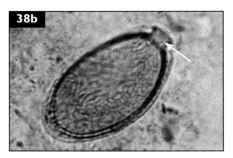

39 i. Osteomyelitis versus a osteolytic neoplasm; more likely osteomyelitis.
ii. Confirm by fine-needle aspirate or open biopsy.
iii. If it is osteomyelitis and amenable to incision and drainage, thorough debridement, microbiological culture and sensitivity testing, followed by an appropriately effective antibiotic administration; if, however, it is found to be an osteolytic bone tumor, the affected entire left fore-limb should be amputated via a high (scapulo-humeral) amputation.

40i. Figure **40a** shows a side-necked turtle, *Pelusios williamsi*. What is your tentative diagnosis?
ii. How would you confirm the diagnosis?
iii. How would you treat this turtle?
iv. What is the prognosis?

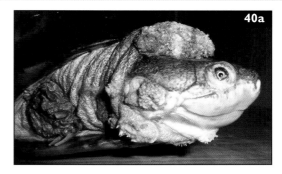

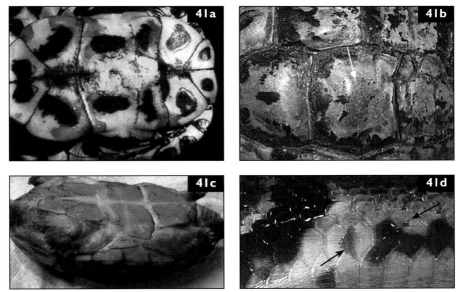

41 Figures **41a–d** illustrate a specific abnormality in a semi-aquatic turtle, a terrestrial tortoise, a musk turtle and a snake.
i. With respect to the snake, arrows point to the lesions. What is your diagnosis?
ii. What tests would you employ to confirm your diagnosis?

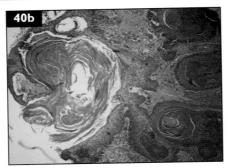

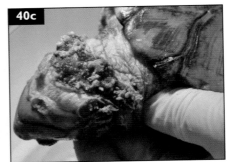

40c Post-treatment photograph. Note the areas of tumor necrosis.

40 i. The turtle has multifocal papillomatous tumors on its head and neck.

ii. The diagnosis can be confirmed via one or more full-thickness excisional biopsies (**40b**).

iii. Because of the multiplicity of lesions on this turtle, several were removed surgically; some specimens were prepared for routine histopathology whilst others were ground aseptically with sterile sand and tissue culture diluent, treated with dilute formalin solution, exposed to unfiltered artificial UV light and then made into an autogenous vaccine, which was injected into the turtle, with booster doses 4 weeks apart.

iv. The prognosis is favorable. This turtle began sloughing its necrotic tumors several weeks after the second dose of autogenous vaccine was injected (**40c**).

41 i. Sub-epidermal hemorrhages.

ii. Microscopic examination of a stained whole blood film to determine the relative presence or absence of thrombocytes.

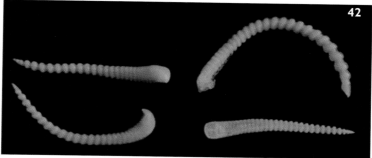

42 The four organisms in Figure 42 are common parasites of snakes. Are they: A, cestodes; B, acanthocephalans; C, pentastomids; D, hookworms?

43 Identify this reptile (43). Is it: A, Gaboon viper; B, tropical rat snake; C, African house snake; D, Central American boa constrictor?

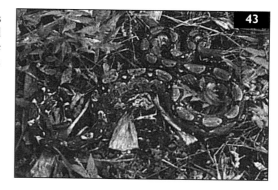

44 Identify this parasitic ovum (44a).

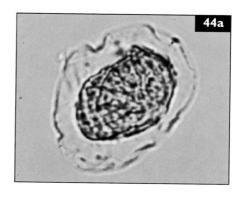

41

42 C, pentastomids.

43 D, a Central American boa constrictor (*Boa constrictor imperator*).

44 It is a cestode (tapeworm) ovum within its membrane. Note the parallel hooklets that are a characteristic feature (**44b**).

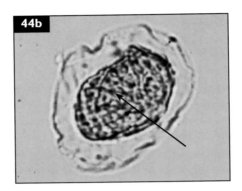

45 Identify this commonly encountered ectoparasite of lizards (45). Is it:
A, trombiculid (grain) mites
B, *Hirstiella trombiidiformis*
C, *Cnimidocoptes* sp.?

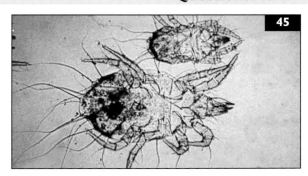

46 What is your impression of this captive Central American boa constrictor (*Boa constrictor imperator*) (46)?

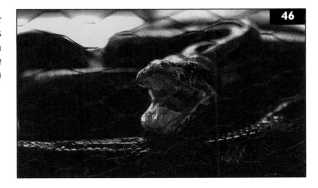

47 Identify the gender of these two Indian star tortoises (*Testudo elegans*) (47a, 47b).

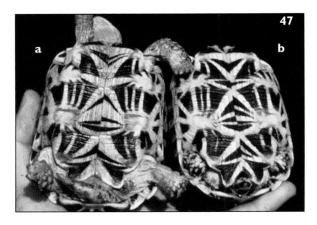

45 A, trombiculid grain mites. These often infest cage litter material.

46 The snake is housed in a chicken wire-covered cage. Furthermore, its ulcerative oral lesions are suggestive that this snake has been sustaining trauma from striking at chicken wire as passersby are within range.

Note: Central American boas (*Boa constrictor imperator*) are not as tractable as their South American cousins (*Boa c. constrictor*) and are *much* more likely to strike out at anyone or anything disturbing them.

47 Figure **47a** is male; note the much larger tail and a concave plastron, which enables it to mount a female without slipping to one side during copulation.

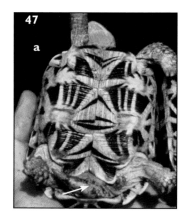

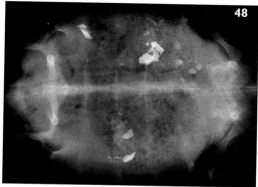

48 i. What is your interpretation/diagnosis of the radiograph of a Texas tortoise (*Xerobates [Gopherus] berlandieri*) shown in Figure 48?
ii. How would you treat this tortoise?

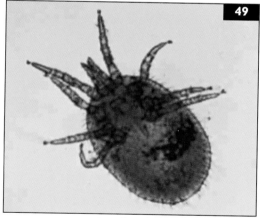

49 Identify this common ectoparasite of snakes and occasionally, lizards (49).

48 i. Multiple metallic foreign bodies within the alimentary system; from their intense radio-opacity, it is likely that they are lead or lead-containing. The laboratory analysis of this turtle's blood lead content was 211 µg/dl (2.1 mg/l), whereas a control Texas tortoise's blood lead content was 25.7 µg/dl (257 µg/l).
ii. Use a bulk laxative and soft diet to aid in the expulsion of the lead fragments from the gastrointestinal tract; also treat the tortoise with the chelating agent, EDTA, intravenously weekly or semi-weekly until the blood lead level diminishes to near normal. Remove waste lead including old lead-painted objects from the environment that is occupied by tortoise(s) or other animals.

49 The organism shown is an adult snake mite, *Ophionyssus natricis*.

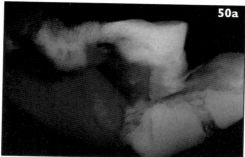

50 Figure 50a is a postmortem radiograph of a California desert tortoise's (*Xerobates [Gopherus] agassizi*) liver after it had been excised from the cadaver. The history obtained from the owner was that the animal had been fed a diet consisting almost entirely of canned or moistened dry dog food and that the tortoise had been on that diet for several years until it was found dead one morning.
i. What is your interpretation/diagnosis of this radiograph adult tortoise's liver?
ii. What is the etiology of this condition?
iii. What is the prognosis for a living animal affected with this condition?
iv. What would you advise the owner to do to avoid this kind of lesion in any other tortoises in this collection?

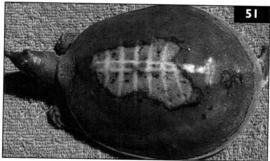

51 i. How would you treat this thermally burned soft-shelled turtle (*Apalone* sp.) (51)?
ii. What special consideration(s) are essential when dealing with soft-shell turtles?

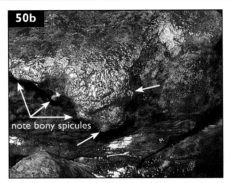

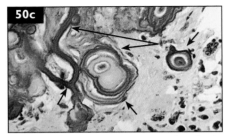

Figure 50b is a photograph of the liver at necropsy and **Figure 50c** a photomicrograph of the liver from this tortoise. Note the newly formed bone in both images.

Figure 50c note osteocytes and multiple cement lines within liver.

50 i. Chronic multifocal to diffuse pathological (dystrophic) ossification and mineralization of the liver; hepatic ossification.
ii. Hypercalcemia secondary to hypervitaminosis-D-3 induced by the feeding of dog food.
iii. The prognosis for a living animal with this condition is guarded to poor because once formed, the ectopic bone is likely to be remain a permanent feature of the hepatic tissue.
iv. The owner should be advised that dog food should not be fed to herbivorous reptiles, particularly when it constitutes the major component of the diet.

51 i. The denuded shell should be cleansed gently with 0.75% chlorhexidine diacetate (or gluconate), air-dried and covered with a liquid plastic antiseptic bandage.
ii. Aquatic soft-shelled turtles must be protected from desiccation of their exquisitely delicate pastrons and carapaces. They are then placed into a shallow tray or bowl containing only a small volume of clean water; then their carapace covered with one or more large gauze sponges so that the edges wick water and, thus, keep the exposed shell surfaces moist. A *bacteriocidal* antibiotic administered parenterally is also recommended. An alternative method of treatment is to cover the exposed tissues with a waterproof plastic antiseptic bandage such as New Skin®. Note: if this product is used, the surfaces upon which it is applied must be oil-free.

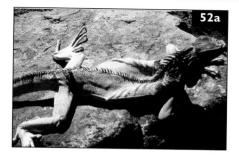
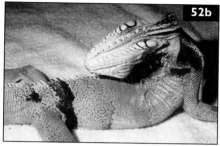
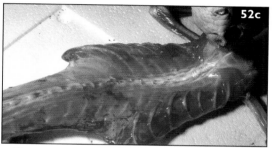

52 Figures **52a–c** illustrate a young green iguana (*Iguana iguana*) with a severe skeletal anomaly.
i. What is your diagnosis of this animal's anatomical anomaly?

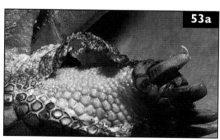
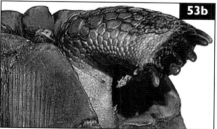

53 Figure **53a** shows a California desert tortoise (*Xerobates [Gopherus] agassizi*) 11 days after receiving an injection of a vitamin. Figure **53b** shows the same tortoise 2 days later.
i. Which vitamin is known to induce this kind of adverse reaction?
ii. How would you treat this condition?
iii. What is the prognosis?

52 i. The iguana had both dorsal and ventral pectus excavatum as well as kyphosis. The additive result of these anomalies was severe compression of the thoracic portion of this iguana's coelomic cavity, leading to eventual cardio-respiratory failure.

53 i. Injectable vitamin A can induce this form or dermatopathy. If extraneous vitamin A is considered to be warranted, administer it orally, not by injection.
ii. In many instances, the tissue will heal after topical application of a thermal burn ointment such as silversulfadiazine. Parenteral broad-spectrum bacteriocidal antibiotic(s) and supportive parenteral fluid therapy are also essential adjunctive therapies.
iii. The prognosis is usually favorable when the patient is treated as indicated above.

54 i. Identify the pink structure lying on this alligator snapping turtle's (*Macrochelys temminckii*) tongue (**54a**).
ii. What is its function?

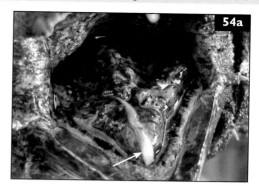

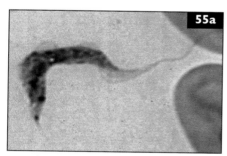

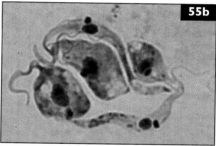

55 Identify these organisms observed in the blood of a Western fence lizard (*Sceloporus occidentalis*) (**55a, b**).

56 i. What is your diagnosis of the radiograph in Figure 56?
ii. What is the etiology of this disorder?
iii. What is the treatment for this disorder?
iv. What is the prognosis for recovery?

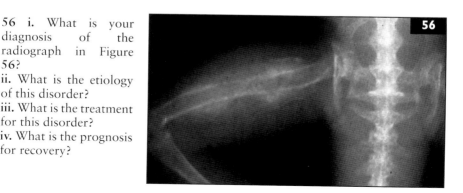

54 i. It is a lingual lure (**54b**).
ii. With their lingual lure, which closely mimics a moving earthworm, submerged alligator snapping turtles entice fish to swim sufficiently close to be caught in their gaping jaws.

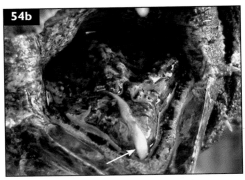

55 *Trypanosoma* sp.

56 i. Secondary nutritional (or renal) hyperparathyroidism.
ii. The etiologies include:
- An overabundance of phosphorus with a concomitant deficiency in calcium in the diet. The ratio of these two essential minerals ideally should be at least Ca:P of 2:1. Metabolic bone disease can also be induced by:
  - o Renal disease that permits the excessive excretion of calcium and the excessive retention of phosphorus.
  - o Parathyroid hormone-secreting parathyroid adenomatous tumors.
  - o Vitamin D-3 deficiency.
iii. Treatment consists of:
- Re-establishing a normal Ca:P ratio of slightly greater than 2:1.
- Oral administration of vitamin D-3, and, in very serious cases, daily administration of calcitonin salmon mucosally, usually in alternating nostrils.
iv. The prognosis is favorable when treated effectively.

57 How would you manage or treat the Meller's chameleon (*Chamaeleo melleri*) with a paralyzed and partially necrotic right hind-limb (57)?

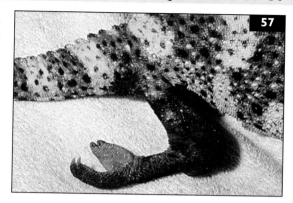

58 i. Identify the two objects revealed during a routine microscopic examination of a reptile's fecal specimen (58).
ii. Is this organism pathogenic?
iii. If you believe that this organism is pathogenic, how would you treat it?

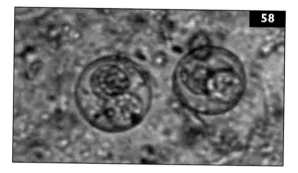

59 i. Identify this animal (59).
ii. What major feature of its life cycle makes it both unique and useful as a biomedical model and study animal?

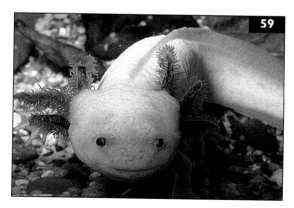

57 Because the limb is paralyzed and partially necrotic, the only practical option is to perform a coxo-femoral disarticulated amputation. With their grasping fore- and hind-limb apposing digits, these arboreal lizards function quite well after losing a limb.

58 i. Sporulated *Isospora* sp.
ii. It is pathogenic.
iii. Treat with any one of the following protozoan parasiticides:
• Metronidazole 20–40 mg/kg, repeated in 14 days.
• Fenbendazole 50 mg/kg, repeated in 14 days.
• Sulfamethoxine 75–90 mg/kg the first day, 40–45 mg/kg for the next 5–6 days.
Make certain that the patient is well hydrated; if necessary, administer parenteral fluids.

59 i. The animal shown is an amelanistic Mexican axolotl, *Ambystoma* sp.
ii. The particularly interesting characteristic of these amphibians is that they do not undergo metamorphosis from a juvenile aquatic larval form into a terrestrial adult form. Thus, these animals attain adulthood and sexual maturity whilst still retaining their juvenile (larval) features. This is termed *neoteny*. Note that this adult still possesses external gills that it employs for respiratory gas exchange.

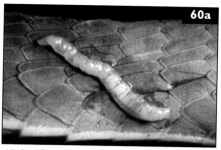
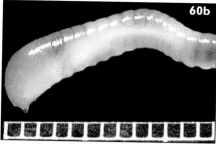

60 i. Identify the parasitic organism that is shown in Figures **60a, 60b**. It was excised from beneath the skin of a tropical vine snake.
ii. Does this parasite utilize an indirect or direct life cycle?
iii. Knowing that a reptile patient is infested with at least several of these parasites, how would you treat it?

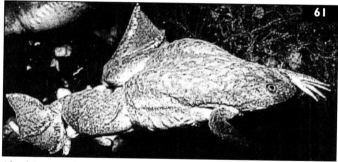

61 i. Identify this popular aquatic amphibian often kept by hobbyists (**61**).
ii. What is a suitable diet for this animal?

60 i. The parasite is a pentastomid. These are not helminths, although they superficially look like 'worms'. They are actually arachnids, distant relatives to spiders and scorpions, that only reveal their four pair of external limbs in their embryonic stage while they are encased within the eggshell.
ii. Pentastomids utilize an indirect life cycle, often a complicated one, involving multiple intermediate hosts before infesting their final or definitive host.
iii. Treatment consists of excising those that can be readily seen as swellings and then administering ivermectin at a dosage of 200 μg/kg (DO NOT ADMINISTER THIS DRUG TO CHELONIANS !!). Note: some pentastomids are zoonotic for humans.

61 i. It is an African clawed frog, *Xenopus laevis*.
ii. These frogs eagerly consume earthworms and appropriately sized fish.

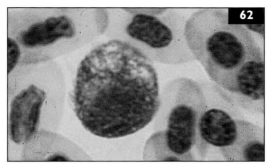

62 i. Identify the cell surrounded by numerous erythrocytes in Figure 62.
ii. What is this cell's function?
iii. If observed in excessive numbers on a stained blood film, what are some plausible diagnostic possibilities?
iv. What are the pale-staining objects within the cytoplasm?
v. Of what are they comprised?

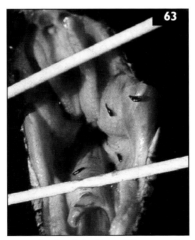

63 Figure 63 shows an anesthetized indigo (*Drymarchon corais*) snake with its mouth being held open. Several black organisms are visible on its oral mucosa.
i. What are these objects?
ii. Do these organisms utilize a direct or indirect life cycle?
iii. How would you treat this snake?
iv. What is the prognosis?
v. How would you prevent this infestation?

62 i. This leukocyte is a plasma cell (plasmacyte). Note its eccentric nucleus, dark blue cytoplasm and pale cytoplasmic inclusions.

ii. These cells are active in synthesizing specific antibodies to specific antigenic substances.

iii. If observed in excessive numbers (plasmacytosis), this can suggest either an antibody response to an antigen, such as an infective organism, or a plasma cell neoplasm (plasmacytoma, multiple myeloma); most (but not invariably all) multiple myelomas are *mono*clonal and, thus, are characterized via electrophoresis; most infections or other antibody responses are *poly*clonal and thus, are often, if not usually, accompanied by a *mixed* leukocytic reaction, which usually includes heterophils, small lymphocytes, eosinophils, azurophils and histiocytic macrophages.

iv. The multiple pale objects (inclusions or areas) are Russell bodies.

v. Russell bodies are thought to be comprised of antibody-rich protein.

63 i. The organisms are renifer trematodes (flukes).

ii. These parasites, like other trematodes, utilize an indirect life cycle, most often involving two or more intermediate hosts such as snails, fish and/or amphibians.

iii. The flukes that are readily accessed are simply picked off with a cotton-tipped applicator. The snake is then administered praziquantel at a dosage of 5–8 mg/kg orally or SC, repeated in 2 weeks.

iv. The prognosis is favorable.

v. Infestation with renifer flukes is easily avoided by feeding only non-infested prey. In this instance, indigo snakes are remarkably broad in their dietary preferences. Thus, they do not *require* the inclusion of amphibians or fish (which are the most frequently trematode-infested prey) in their diet.

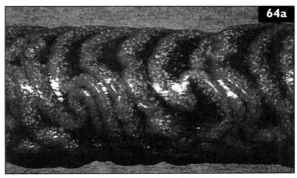

64 Figure **64a** is that of a snake's kidney revealed during a necropsy examination.
i. What is your diagnosis?

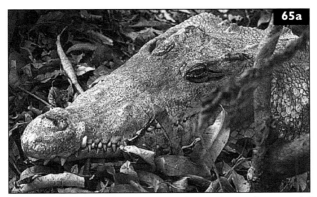

65 i. Identify the reptile in Figure **65a**. Is it: A, a caiman; B, a gavial (or gharial);
C, a crocodile; D, an alligator?
ii. On what specific criterion or criteria did you make your choice?

64 i. Visceral (renal) gout. Note the myriad number of punctate grayish foci, which are accumulations of crystalline urates (gouty tophi [**64b**]).

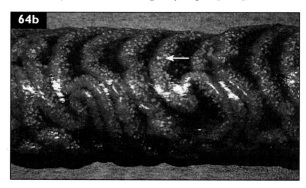

65 i. C, an American crocodile (*Crocodyus acutus*).
ii. There are two major criteria upon which to base your answer. Most, but not all crocodiles possess a narrow snout, whereas alligators and caiman have a much broader snout. There is, however, a broad-nosed crocodile. A second criterion is that a crocodile's fourth mandibular tooth fits into a shallow groove in the upper jaw, whereas the fourth mandibular teeth of alligators and caiman are accommodated in pits in the upper arcade of teeth and, thus are usually not readily seen when the animals have their mouths closed. In this image, you can clearly see the fourth lower mandibular tooth (**65b**). Gavials (gharials) have greatly elongated and very narrow upper and lower jaws.

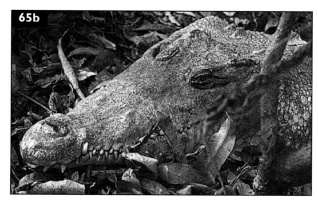

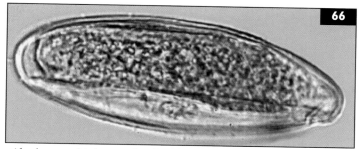

66 i. Identify the merthiolate-stained organism shown in Figure 66.
ii. Is it pathogenic?
iii. If pathogenic, how would you treat a reptilian patient infested with this organism?

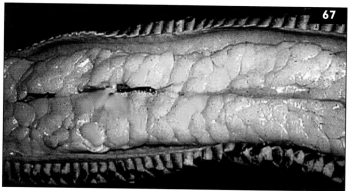

67 Identify the pale yellow-pink tissue within the body wall of the python shown in the necropsy photograph (67).

66 i. It is an embryonated oxyurid (pinworm) ovum.

ii. It is pathogenic and is often implicated in both intussusceptions and colorectal prolapses, especially in lizards.

iii. These helminthes are readily and effectively treated with any of several antihelminth parasiticides, such as pyrantel at a dosage of 5.0 mg/kg, or febendazole at a dosage of 50 mg/kg repeated in 2 and again at 4 weeks.

Note: some authorities have proposed that oxyurid helminths participate as a normal constituent of digestion in herbivorous animals; others disagree. Parasite-free lizards appear to thrive without being burdened with these helminths. Nevertheless, it is advisable to rid a reptilian or amphibious patient of its parasites.

67 The tissue is adipose tissue comprising intracoelomic fat bodies.

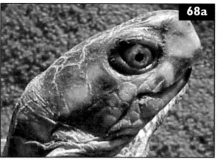
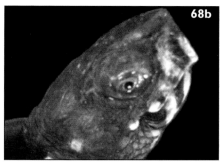

68 i. In Figures **68a, 68b** of two North American box turtles, which is a male and which is a female?
ii. On what criterion did you decide your answer?

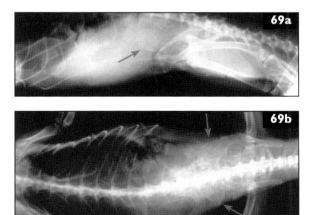

69 Lateral (**69a**) and dorso-ventral (**69b**) radiographs of a mature female green iguana (*Iguana iguana*) are shown. While having its coelomic contents palpated during a physical examination, the iguana was found to possess firm, distinctly irregular lumpy kidneys. The iguana's history revealed that the vegetable diet was supplemented three times weekly with monkey biscuits and a commercial calcium–vitamin D-3 product.
i. Examine these two radiographs, particularly those portions indicated by arrows. What is your interpretation/diagnosis of the lesions?
ii. What is the etiology of these lesions?
iii. What is the prognosis for this condition in this lizard?
iv. What would you advise the owner to do to avoid this condition in the future with other iguanas in the collection?

68 i. The female is shown in Figure **68a**, the male in Figure **68b**.

ii. One useful criterion is the color of the iris; the male's is red, the female's is yellow-gold. This characteristic applies to only some species; thus, it is is useful, but it is not universal across the entire genus *Terrapene*.

69 i. Dystrophic mineralization–ossification of the peripheral renal capsules.

ii. The *most likely* etiology for this soft-tissue mineralization is hypercalcemia secondary to hypervitaminosis D-3.

iii. The prognosis is guarded to unfavorable because once formed the new bone is permanent.

iv. The owner should be advised to reduce the amount of both calcium and, especially, vitamin D-3 supplementation.

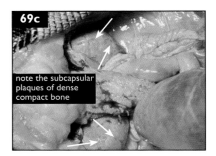

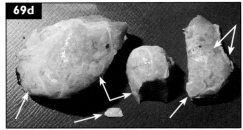

69d Arrows point to bony sub- and intracapsular plaques

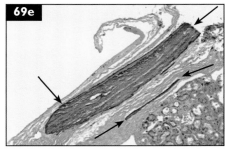

Figures 69c–69e show the gross pathology and histopathology of these lesions.
69e Note the plaques of ectopic ossification embedded within the tissues of the renal cortex (black arrows).

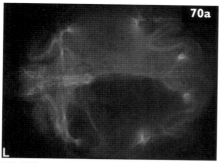 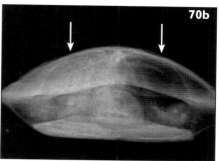

70 What is your diagnosis of the problem in the radiographic images shown in Figures **70a, 70b** of a North American painted turtle (*Chrysemys picta*)?

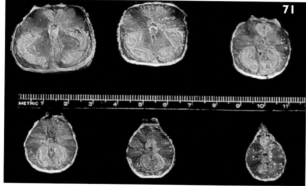

71 Figure **71** shows whole mount cross-sections of the tail of a caiman (*Caiman crocodilus*), a South and Central American crocodilian. Numerous yellow-orange lesions are readily seen in the tissues that have been exposed. These lesions possess a distinctly dry, waxy appearance and a slight odor of fish.
i. What is your diagnosis?
ii. What is the etiology of this condition?
iii. How can it be prevented?

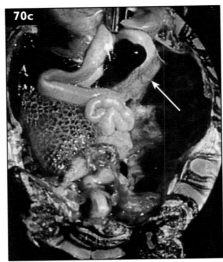

70 Unilateral (left) pulmonary collapse/loss of aeration. Figure 70c illustrates the gross appearance of this turtle's left lung. The arrow points to the complete consolidation of the entire left lungfield that was found to be affected by diffuse chronic granulomatous pneumonia.

71 i. These orange, dry lesions that have a fish-like odor are characteristic of steatitis (panniculitis), the chronic inflammation of fatty tissue.
ii. The etiology of this condition is a relative deficiency in vitamin E that is often induced by the chronic ingestion of foods containing rancid long-chain fatty acids.
iii. Steatitis can be prevented by feeding *fresh* foods, especially those that are rich in fats and oils. Feeding a varied diet also helps in preventing this acquired nutritional condition and is recommended.

72 The following is a portion of the laboratory analysis of blood taken from a moribund wild-caught adult female Pacific pond turtle (*Actremys marmorata*) that died 11 days after she was presented for examination and evaluation after her sudden onset of profound lethargy.

WBC	8,750/mm^3 (8.75 × 10^9/l)
Lymphocytes	29%
Heterophils	42%
Azurophils	19%
Monocytes	7%
Basophils	3%
Erythrocytes	2,900,000 /mm^3 (2.9 × 10^{12}/l)
Total protein	8.5 mg/dl (85 mg/l)
Globulin	5.7 mg/dl (57 mg/l)
Albumin:globulin ratio	2.03:1
Glucose	842.0 mg/dl (46.7 mmol/l)

i. What is your interpretation of the turtle's blood analysis and what is your diagnosis?
ii. How do you explain the blood proteins?

72 i. The WBC and red blood cells are essentially normal. The differential counts are slightly but, not significantly skewed towards heterophilia and azurophilia. The total protein is elevated and a portion of that elevation probably can be attributed to dehydration, but not in its entirety. Certainly, the globulin fraction is substantially elevated and this may be of great significance. The single most significant abnormality in the laboratory report is the elevated blood glucose level. Clearly, this turtle was diabetic at the time of its demise.

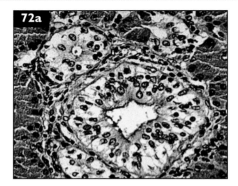

ii. Considering the combined findings of severe hyperglycemia and as well as hyperglobinemia, a logical conclusion is an autoimmune pancreatic isleitis that selectively destroyed the islets of insulin-secreting beta cells. Histopathology of this turtle's visceral tissues revealed that its pancreatic islets were severely infiltrated by plasma cells, leaving only a few relatively normal and non-infiltrated. This case confirms not only the provisional diagnosis, but also the great value of routine diagnostic histopathology (72a–72c). Thus, the hyperglobinemia that was associated with the hyperglycemia is explained. Although this turtle was an adult, its clinical course and etiology are similar to Type I or juvenile, diabetes in humans.

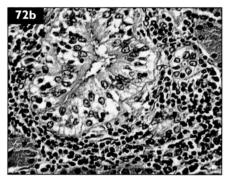

72a A relatively normal islet of Langerhans. There are, however numerous plasma cells at the interface of the islet with the surrounding pancreatic exocrine tissues. H&E stain, × 430 magnification.

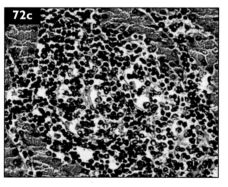

72b A moderately infiltrated islet exhibiting greater infiltration by plasma cells. H&E stain, × 430 magnification.

72c A severely infiltrated islet, representative of the majority of those observed in this turtle's pancreas. Note that most of the cells comprising the islet have been destroyed, leaving very few behind to function and secrete insulin. H&E stain, × 430 magnification.

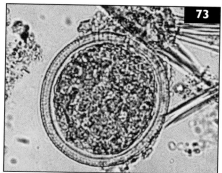

73 i. Identify this object observed during the microscopic examination of the feces of a Nile monitor (*Varanus niloticus*) (73).
ii. Would you treat this large lizard for this organism?
iii. If you would treat, what would you administer, how and by what route?

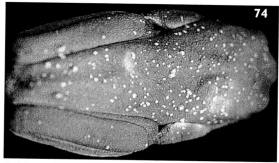

74 Figure **74** of this red-eyed tree frog (*Agalychnis callidryas*) was recorded in the rain forest of Central America. This was one of several recently captured amphibians.
i. What is your interpretation/diagnosis of this frog's integumentary condition?
ii. How would you investigate this outbreak of skin disease in this group of frogs?
iii. What advice would you give to the owner of these frogs, pending a definitive diagnosis, to help reduce the chances for further spread of an infectious agent among the remaining healthy frogs?

73 i. The object is an embryonated ascarid ovum.

ii. This is a parasite and, thus, the patient *should* be treated.

iii. A patient infested with ascarid nematodes can be treated effectively by the oral administration of any of the following anthelminthics: pyrantel pamoate, fenbendazole, ivermectin, etc. Often the dosage can be delivered by inserting/injecting it into a prey item. If the monitor lizard is large or fractious, ivermectin can be administered via an injection either SC or IM.

74 i. The multifocal raised white epidermal lesions *could* be of bacterial, fungal or parasitic etiology. Because there were multiple cases within the recently captured frogs, it is likely that the commonality of this disease outbreak is due to an infectious organism, most likely bacterial or mycotic (fungal), perhaps both, as a mixed infection.

ii. The most direct means for formulating an accurate diagnosis is to select several representative frogs with typical dermal lesions and perform microbiological culture and sensitivity testing (including mycological culture), touch-preparation cytology and histopathology employing special fungal staining techniques.

iii. The best advice would be to isolate the healthy frogs from those that display epidermal lesions. A strict quarantine, hygiene and culling of affected individuals is essential in such outbreaks. The histopathology revealed multifocal bacterial dermatitis.

75 Figures 75a, 75b show the tail region of a soft-shelled turtle (*Apalone* sp.) with a recently acquired lesion.

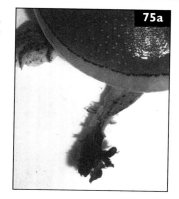
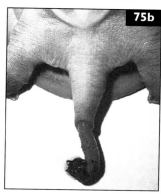

i. What is your interpretation/ diagnosis of this turtle's condition?
ii. How would you manage or treat this patient?
iii. What do you think was the etiology of this condition?
iv. What is your prognosis?

76 Identify the turtle in Figure 76.

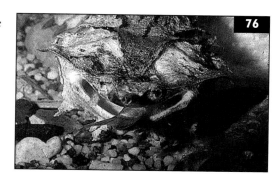

77 Identify the parasitic ovum shown in Figure 77a. Is it:
A, a pentastomid
B, an acanthacephalan
C, a cestode
D, a trematode?

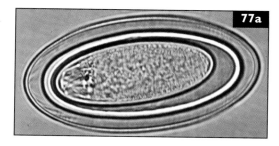

71

75 i. This turtle's penis has been traumatized, leaving its end shredded.
ii. The penis is (1) severely damaged and (2) flaccid, thus effectively forfeiting it's effective use in the future as a copulatory organ. The penis should be amputated.
iii. The most likely etiology for this lesion is the turtle's tank mates mistaking the tumescent organ for a worm or other prey item and inflicting multiple bites on it before the turtle could withdraw it.
iv. The prognosis for survival and normal life expectancy is favorable. However, this turtle's future as a sire has been forestalled.

76 Mata mata turtle (*Chelys fimbriata*).

77 B, an acanthacephalan (thorny-headed worm). Note the thick, multilayered shell and the thorny hooklets at one end of the embryo (**77b**).

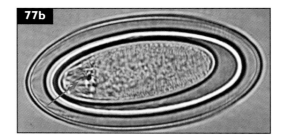

78 i. Identify the ovum in Figure 78. Is it:
A, *Dasymetra* sp.; B, *Mesocestoides* sp.; C,
Ascaris sp.; D, *Capillaria* sp.?
ii. Upon what criterion did you rely to make
your identification?

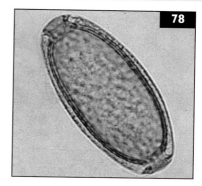

79 What is your interpretation
of this snake's ocular
appearance (79)?

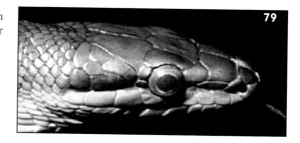

80 i. Identify this commonly kept lizard (80a).
ii. What is its gender?

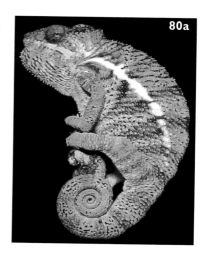

78 i. D, *Capillaria* sp.
ii. The ova of *Capillaria* are characterized by a plug-like operculum at each end. Note: the ova of trematodes (flukes) are similar but have only a single operculum at one end.

79 The tertiary spectacle covering the cornea appears slightly opaque or 'milky'. This change in appearance occurs a few days prior to normal shedding or ecdysis. A day or two prior to actual ecdysis the corneas clear. During these few days preparatory to ecdysis most snakes do not feed.

80 i. It is a panther chameleon, *Furcifer pardalis*.
ii. It is a male. The female of this species is drab in her coloration. Also, the left hemipenial bulge can be seen in **80b**.

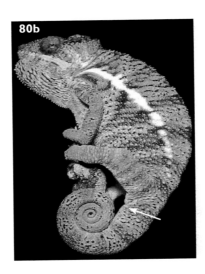

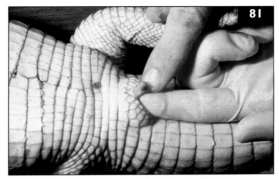

81 Figure **81** shows a juvenile American alligator (*Alligator mississippiensis*) being restrained for examination. Identify the small structure at the tip of the examiner's finger.

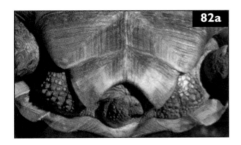

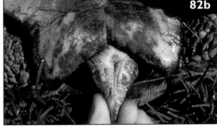

82 Identify the gender of the following sets of paired chelonians: adult California desert tortoises (*Xerobates [Gopherus] agassizi*) (**82a, b**), adult musk turtles (*Sternotherus* sp.) (**82c**).

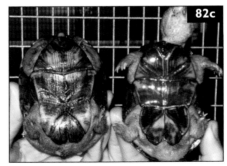

81 The structure is the penis. Note: although earlier texts state that male crocodilians lack an erectile penis, one can see from this image that these animals do possess one; however, it is diminutive.

82 In both sets the female is on the left; the male is on the right.

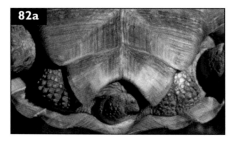

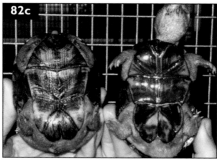

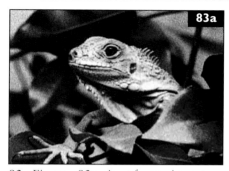

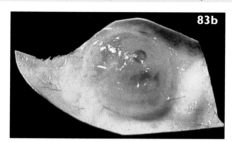

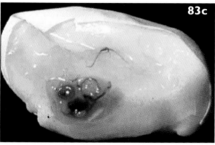

83 Figure 83a is of an immature 7-month-old female green iguana (*Iguana iguana*) that had been housed by herself until she was placed with a male iguana for a few weeks, after which, she was again isolated in a cage by herself. When she was approximately 2.5 years old, she began to deposit eggs, none of which hatched. When she was slightly over 3.5 years old, she produced a clutch of 11 eggs. Two of those eggs were submitted for examination (83b, 83c).

i. How do you explain how a female iguana that has not had contact with a male of her species could have produced embryonated eggs so long after any opportunity for her to mate? Which of the following offers the most logical explanation: A, parthenogenesis ('virgin birth'; 'immaculate conception'); B, 'immaculate *deception*' (she actually must have been bred more recently); C, *amphigonia retardata* (she stored sperm until they were used to fertilize her ova)?

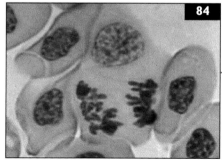

84 What is your interpretation of the large cell in Figure 84?

83 i. C, *amphigonia retardata*. Some reptiles can store viable spermatozoa within crypt-like spaces in the walls of their oviducts for prolonged periods of time, often several years. During that time, the sperm are nourished by the secretions elaborated by the cells lining those crypts.

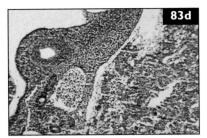

AUTHOR'S NOTE: although some authorities have written that iguana eggs do not commence embryonic development until the fertilized eggs are exposed to atmospheric oxygen, this case refutes that claim. Although the eggs shown here were deposited on the day that they were opened and examined, histological examination of the embryos revealed relatively well advanced organogenesis and even clear evidence of early cellular immunity. Figures 83d–h provide ample evidence of early intestinal, renal, hepatic, cardiovascular, and even neural development in those two iguana embryos.

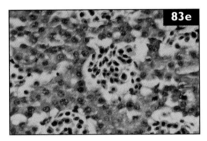

83d Histological section of early iguana embryo showing gut on the left and liver on the right.

83e Photomicrograph of embryonic hepatocellular (liver) tissue.

83f Photomicrograph of embryonic cardiovascular tissue.

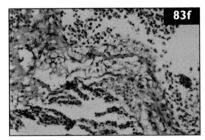

83g Photomicrograph of embryonic renal tissue. Note the glomerular and renal tubular structures.

83h Photomicrograph of embryonic brain tissue.

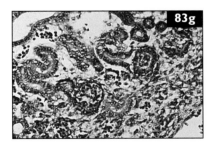

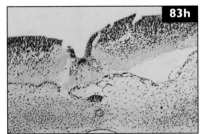

84 Dedifferentiation metaphase mitotic division of a previous hemoglobin-containing mature erythrocyte. The cell immediately above it is in early prophase and is also about to divide.

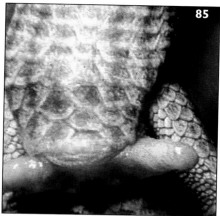

85 Identify the two objects that are protruding from the anal area of a North American alligator lizard (*Elgaria* sp.) (85).

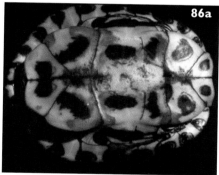

86 i. What is your interpretation of this red-eared slider turtle's (*Trachemys scripta elegans*) medical condition (86a)?
ii. How would you confirm your diagnosis?
iii. What is a likely etiology for inducing this condition?

85 The two objects are hemipenes. These are twin copulatory organs or phalli and are a characteristic of male snakes and lizards.

86 i. This turtle exhibits multiple sub-epidermal hemorrhages, perhaps thrombocytopenic purpura.
ii. Microscopic examination of a stained blood film, looking for the presence and number of thrombocytes.
iii. There are many etiologies for the induction of thrombocytopenia. These include, but are *not* limited to: bacterial and viral infections, autoimmune hemolytic anemia, some hemic parasitic infestations, severe acute anemia, hemorrhage and DIC. Because reptiles under severe acute erythrocytic loss can dedifferentiate and transform some of their mature thrombocytes into erythrocytes, the diminishment of the existing thrombocyte pool can, under some conditions, lead to acute thrombocytopenia and spontaneous hemorrhage (**86b, 86c**)

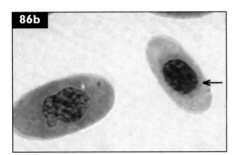 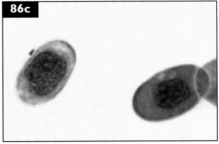

86b, c Snake erythrocytes dedifferentiating and transforming into hemoglobin-containing erythrocytes. Benzindine peroxidase stain, × 360 original magnification.

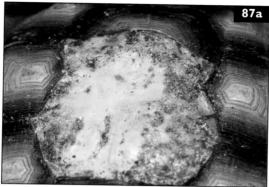

87 Figure **87a** shows an African spurred tortoise (*Geochelone sulcata*) with an epidermal lesion on its central-posterior carapacial scutes (plates).
i. What are some provisional (tentative) diagnoses?
ii. What tests or procedures would you order or apply to aid in confirming your diagnosis?
iii. How would you treat this tortoise for this condition?
iv. What is the prognosis?

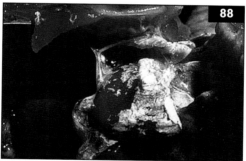

88 Figure **88** was recorded during a necropsy examination of a California desert tortoise (*Xerobates [Gopherus] agassizi*).
i. What is your interpretation of the peri- and epicardial tissues revealed?

87 i. Provisional diagnoses include fungal (mycotic), bacterial, or parasitic invasion of the keratinized scutes with undermining of the hard keratin such that several scutes have been lost entirely leaving the subepithelial tissues exposed. **ii.** Diagnostic tests should include microbiological culture and sensitivity testing, cytological examination of the lesion and any exudates of cellular debris, and a biopsy if these procedures suggest one is necessary. **iii.** Effective treatment is predicated upon an accurate diagnosis. In this case, the lesion above was found to be induced by an infestation with mites. (As of the date of writing, the taxonomic classification of these mites has yet to be established.)

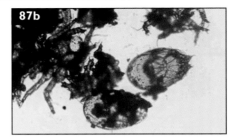

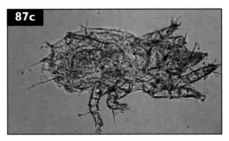

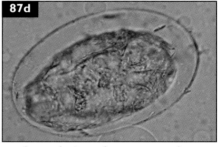

Thus, treatment with a *topical* application of ivermectin preparation was used after a gentle, yet thorough debridement of all undermined carapacial scutes. The topical spray was prepared by mixing 1.0 ml large animal invermectin stock solution in a 3.0 ml syringe with 2.0 ml propylene glycol, then adding those two ingredients after they have been mixed thoroughly, to 1.0 liter of distilled or deionized water. This was applied topically as a fine spray twice weekly for several months in order to ensure that any mites hatching from eggs would be eradicated before they could mature.

AUTHOR'S NOTE: because of its recognized toxicity for chelonians, ivermectin is not recommended for turtles, terrapins or tortoises. However, when it is applied topically as described above, it has proven to be both safe and effective. It should NOT be administered via injection or orally in chelonians! When applied topically, it MUST be diluted as described above. Figures **87b–d** show the mites that were recovered from the lesions.

87b Uncleared adult and nymphal mites.

87c Cleared adult mite from carapacial lesion.

87d Embryonated mite ovum recovered from an active lesion.

88 i. Visceral gout, secondary to hyperuricemia. The white material on these tissues are salts of uric acid.

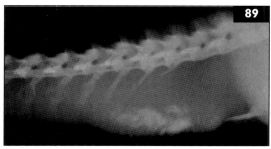

89 Identify the radio-opaque tissue in the radiograph in Figure 89 of an adult male monitor lizard (*Varanus* sp.).

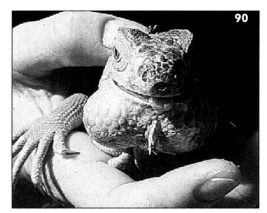

90 i. What is your diagnosis of this green iguana's (*Iguana iguana*) condition (90)?
ii. What is the etiology?
iii. What is the treatment?
iv. What is the prognosis?

89 Mineralized hemipenes. The opposite one cannot be seen clearly in this view. Whether this is a normal condition or an example of dystrophic mineralization is not understood because it occurs in several species of large varanids. When it is observed, the affected males appear to be fully capable of erecting their hemipenes.

90 i. Nutritional secondary hyperparathyroidism.
ii. The etiology is a gross imbalance between the calcium and phosphorus content of the diet, with the phosphorus far in excess and deficient calcium. Additionally, primary hyperparathyroidism and renal disease leading to phosphorus retention and calcium loss can also induce this disease.
iii. Treatment is directed toward improving the diet by restoring the Ca:P ratio to *at least* 2:1, and supplementing the diet with vitamin D-3. In severe cases, calcitonin salmon is administered as a nasal instillation once daily.
iv. The prognosis is favorable when treated aggressively.

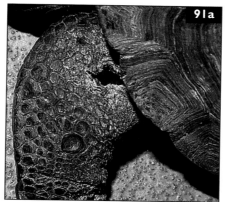

91 Figure **91a** shows an adult male California desert tortoise's (*Xerobates* [*Gopherus*] *agassizi*) left fore-limb.
i. What are some logical provisional diagnoses?
ii. What diagnostic tests would you employ to confirm your diagnosis?
iii. How would you treat/manage this tortoise?

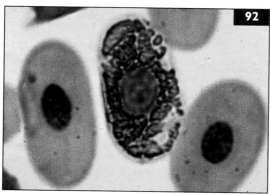

92 What is your interpretation/diagnosis of the erythrocyte in the center of Figure 92?

91 i. Diagnostic possibilities are an inflammatory process, such as an abscess or pyogranulomata following a traumatic wound; a destructive tumor; hematoma; or obstructive vascular process.

ii. Essential diagnostic procedures include plain-film radiography (**91b**), cytology (**91c**), biopsy, microbiological culture and antibiotic sensitivity testing.

Because of the nature of this infection, the entire left fore-limb was amputated and the tortoise made an uneventful recovery. The tortoise soon learned to ambulate on three legs without turning in circles. Note the dense fibrous connective tissue surrounding the inflammation in this operative specimen of the left fore-limb (**91d**).

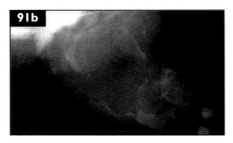

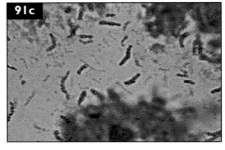

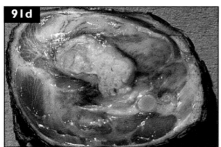

91b Note the extensive osteolysis and new bone formation in this radiograph.
91c Fite's acid-fast stain of exudate recovered from biopsy and mycobacterial culture from biopsy specimen. Note characteristic beaded appearance of these acid-fast micro-organisms.

92 The erythrocyte is infected with the malarial parasite, *Plasmodium* sp.

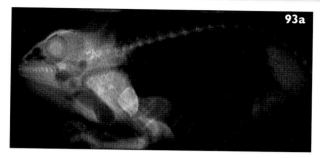

93 i. What is your diagnosis of these lateral (**93a**) and dorso-ventral (**93b**) radiographic views of a male veiled chameleon (*Chamaeleo calyptratus*)? The history of this lizard's captive husbandry revealed that it was fed a daily diet of crickets dusted with a calcium powder that was supplemented with vitamin D-3.

ii. What was the etiology of this lizard's medical condition?

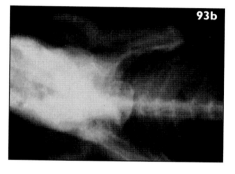

94 Figure **94** is a radiograph of an adult female Texas tortoise (*Xerobates [Gopherus] berlanderi*) that was presented distressed and with tenesmus. She had been straining for at least 3 days prior to examination and evaluation.

i. What is your diagnosis?

ii. How would you treat/manage this animal?

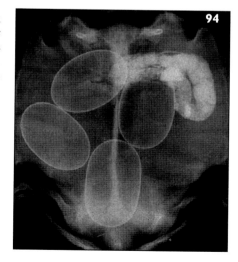

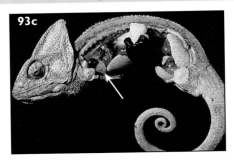

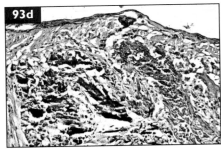

93d Note the severely mineralized myocardial tissues.

93 i. Calcinosis cordis. Figure **93c** was recorded during the necropsy examination (white arrow is pointing to the heart) and a photomicrograph of the histological lesions is shown in Figure **93d**.
ii. Hypercalcemia and dystrophic mineralization secondary to hypervitaminosis D-3.

94 i. Four shelled eggs are seen within the coelom; the most caudal appears to have a cross-sectional diameter that should permit it to pass unobstructed through the pelvic canal. The two most cranial eggs give the impression that they may be exerting extramural pressure upon the stomach and intestines.
ii. Because the eggs do not reveal any anomalous features, the most logical course of action to follow is to prime the tortoise with an appropriate dose of calcium gluconate via an intravenous or subcutaneous injection at a dosage of 10–50 mg/kg, wait for an hour, and then inject oxytocin at an IM dosage of 1–2 U per 100 g body weight. If necessary, repeat oxytocin in 2–4 hours. In most instances this method of treatment for dystocia is successful. If the eggs are not delivered within 6–8 hours, perform a generous transplastron plastotomy incision that provides adequate exposure to the egg-containing oviduct(s); followed by closure of the salpingotomy, rectus musculature and plastron incisions with an external fiberglass and epoxy resin patch.

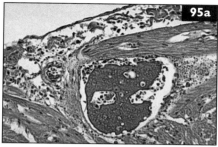

95a Myocardium.

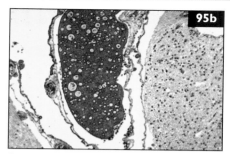

95b Brain.

95 Figures **95a, 95b** demonstrate instances of yolk lipid embolism in several different reptiles.
i. How does this material reach these various distant anatomical sites?

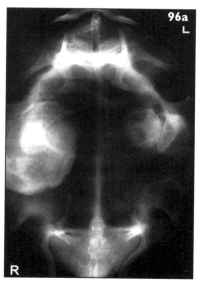

96 What is your interpretation or diagnosis of this of this tortoise's medical condition (**96a**)?

95 i. The yolk lipid escapes from one or more ruptured ova or fractured eggs within the coelomic cavity, through tears in the oviductal wall. The yolk tends to induce a cellular inflammatory response; it is at least partially phagocytized by tissue histiocytes and, perhaps, by other wandering mononuclear leukocytes that gain entry to the vascular system and are then carried to widely separated sites via the circulation. Once they reach blood vessels that are too narrow to permit them to pass, they form emboli that obstruct blood flow beyond the point of obstruction; when they disintegrate into smaller pieces these fragments can travel further to more distant sites where again, they may block vascular flow.

96 There are three radio-opaque objects within the coelomic cavity of this tortoise (96b). The large one in the right lateral mid-coelom and the smaller round one in the left lateral mid-coelom are consistent with mineralized urocystoliths. The object just lateral to the bladder stone on the left side appears to be attached to the inner pillar-like 'bridge' that connects the ventral plastron to the dorsolateral carapace that comprise the tortoise' shell. At surgery, the two urocystoliths were removed through a generous rectangular flap incision and urocystotomy. Lastly, the third object was explored and found to be a bony cyst that, upon opening and evacuation of its contents, contained a porcupine quill. The tortoise made an uneventful recovery after surgery.

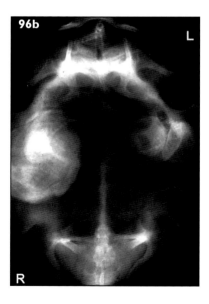

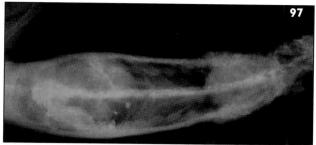

97 i. What is your interpretation/diagnosis of the sub-adult green iguana's (*Iguana iguana*) medical condition displayed in Figure 97?
ii. What is its etiology/pathogenesis?
iii. How would you treat this patient?
iv. How would you prevent it?

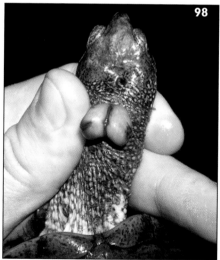

98 i. What is your interpretation/diagnosis of lesion on the dorsum of this turtle's neck (98a)?
ii. How would you confirm your diagnosis?

97 i. Rickets, one of many forms of nutritionally- and/or captive environmentally-induced osteopathic diseases affecting reptiles.

ii. Dietary vitamin D-3 deficiency and/or lack of adequate natural or artificial UV (UVB) irradiation are usually involved in this condition. Hypovitaminosis D-3 induces hypocalcemia, which leads to nutritional secondary hyperparathyroidism.

iii. Administer oral vitamin D-3 and calcium gluconate. Provide a source of natural or appropriate artificial UVB irradiation (see below); improve diet to include food items rich in calcium and relatively low in phosphorus, with a Ca:P ratio of 2:1 or greater.

iv. Feed a diet consisting of green leafy vegetables that are naturally rich in calcium and modest in phosphorus and provide access to natural or artificial UVB irradiation with a wavelength of 280–335 nm.

98 i. Osteoma cutis (**98b**).

ii. Excisional biopsy. Osteomata are characteristically comprised of dense compact bone with a variable amount of less dense cancellous bone. Therefore, it may be difficult to insert a biopsy needle into their deeper portions. Thus, because they are usually discrete lesions, they are readily amenable to simple excision, rather than needle biopsy.

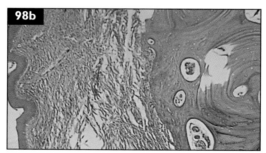

98b Photomicrograph of osteoma cutis. To the left is the cutaneous surface, overlying a loosely arranged dermis comprising collagenous fibrous connective tissue, and the dense compact bone and open spaces of cancellous bone containing sparse bone marrow. Note the multiple concentric cement lines in the compact bone.

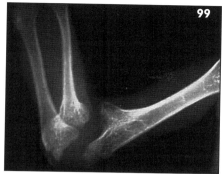

99 Figure 99 is a radiograph of a mature male green iguana's (*Iguana iguana*) left fore-limb. The iguana had been reluctant to use its limb for 6 weeks prior to this radiograph being recorded.
i. What is your diagnosis?
ii. How would you confirm the diagnosis?
iii. How would you treat or manage this patient?
iv. What is the prognosis?

100 Firm but gentle digital palpation of this chameleon's perineal region revealed firm, unyielding swellings (100a, 100b).
i. What is your diagnosis of this chameleon's medical condition?
ii. How would you treat this patient?
iii. What is the etiology of this condition?
iv. What recommendation(s) would you make to the owner of this lizard?

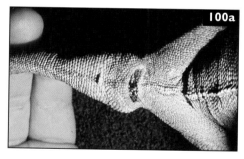

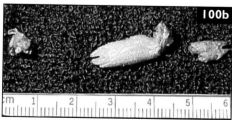

99 i. Provisional diagnoses include an inflammatory process such as osteomyelitis, rheumatoid arthritis or neoplasia.

ii. The diagnosis can be confirmed by fine-needle aspirate biopsy. If the lesion is related to an infectious agent, treatment is directed toward resolving it with antibiotic therapy; if it is shown to be an autoimmune inflammation, treatment would be via anti-inflammatory and analgesic agents to control pain. Note there is little soft-tissue swelling and regeneration of new bone associated with this lesion; while not necessarily confirmatory, the absence of these characteristics suggests that the lesion is not neoplastic. If it were strictly inflammatory, one would expect soft-tissue swelling to be more prominent.

iii. Treatment for a lesion such as this depends upon verification of the diagnosis. In this case, the confirmed diagnosis was osteomyelitis. The radial–humeral joint was opened and carefully curetted. Specimens were collected for microbiological culture and sensitivity testing, then the site was lavaged with 0.75% chlorhexidine diacetate to remove any residual infected and devitalized tissue. This was followed by insertion of an appropriate antibiotic-soaked intra-articular pack, which was changed daily.

iv. The prognosis depends upon the response to the conservative treatment above; if the affected limb does not react satisfactorily and heal, it might necessitate amputation in order to prevent widespread dissemination of the infection.

100 i. Inspissated smegma (seminal) plugs.

ii. A small volume of an oily ointment is instilled into the perihemipenial sulci and gently massaged to distribute it thoroughly; afterward, the individual plugs are massaged toward the cloacal opening until they can be grasped and removed.

iii. These lizards are native to relatively humid environments. When they are housed in captivity with low humidity the smegma that is usually lost during normal copulatory activity accumulates.

iv. The captive environmental humidity should closely mimic natural conditions. Also, this condition is more often encountered in solitary males that do not have an opportunity to copulate. If possible house males with conspecific females.

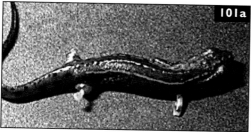

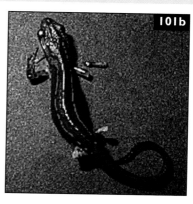

101 Figures **101a**, **101b** show a newt that has suffered autoamputation of three of its four appendicular limb segments.
i. What is the most likely etiology for this striking condition?
ii. Is it possible for this animal to regenerate its missing limbs?

102 In Figure **102** black arrows point to brown objects scattered in the background tissues of this biopsy specimen of a salamander (*Ambystoma* sp.).
i. Identify these objects.
ii. Are they pathogenic?

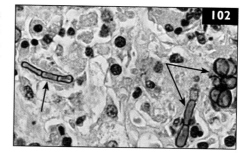

103 Identify the object in the radiograph of a green iguana (*Iguana iguana*) in Figure **103** delineated by the two arrows.

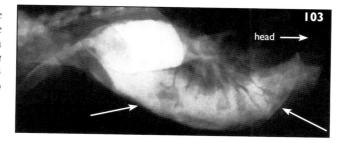

101 i. Any of several Gram-negative pathogenic bacteria can induce this autoamputation of extremities; the most common are *Aeromonas* sp., *Pseudomonas* sp. and *Klebsiella* sp.
ii. Yes. Newts and salamanders can regenerate missing body parts and retain this ability throughout their lifespan, although it may diminish with age and previous regeneration(s) of lost parts. This ability is due to activation of resting stem cells. However, in cases such as this one, the infection is likely to cause further tissue loss – and death – unless it is halted by natural or artificial antibiosis.

102 i. The brown objects are septated elements of the pigmented fungal organism, *Homodendrum* sp.
ii. Yes, they *are* pathogenic fungal organisms and often induce mycotic granulomatous inflammatory lesions. These organisms are zoonotic for humans.

103 The structure is the sacculated colon. Its radiodensity is a consequence of the ingesta and fluid that it contains.

104 In Figure **104a** a North American leopard frog (*Rana pipiens*) is shown unable to use its right hind-limb. There was no history or likelihood of trauma affecting this frog.
i. What common infectious organism do you suspect might be inducing this neurological sign?
ii. What tests or procedures would you employ to aid in your diagnosis?

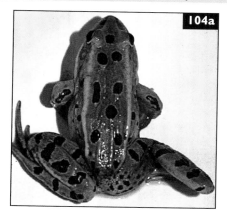

105 i. What is your diagnosis of this gray-banded king snake (*Lampropeltis mexicana alterna*) with a swelling in the region of its stomach (**105a–c**)?
ii. What is the etiological organism?
iii. How would your confirm your diagnosis?

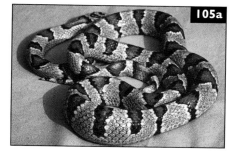

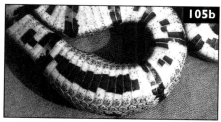

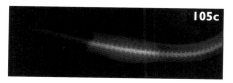

104 i. Infection with the mycotic microorganism, *Batrachochytrium dendrobatidis* must be considered as a possible etiological agent.

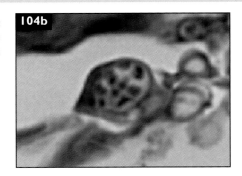

ii. Useful tests include:
- Cytology of skin scrapings or swabs and histopathological examination of tissue sections, searching for the typical cysts containing endospores of the organism (**104b, 104c**).
- Polymerase chain reaction (PCR) of exudates using specific probes directed against this pathogen.

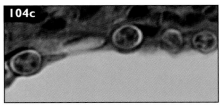

As mentioned in the Preface to this book, in late 2014 a second species of the fungal pathogen, *Batrachochytrium salamandrivorans*, was reported in salamanders and newts in Europe. This organism appears to have arrived with tailed amphibians shipped from Southeast Asia.

104b, c Histopathological examination of stained thin sections of the integument and mucus from the leopard frog. The circular objects contain irregular dark-staining endospores, which when released become motile and infective zoospores (**104d**).

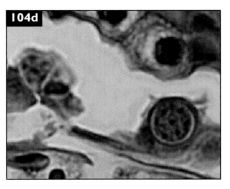

105 i. Cryptosporidiosis.
ii. *Cryptosporidium serpentis*.
iii. The diagnosis can be confirmed with the cytological examination of stained gastric washings and/or stained histological biopsy specimens of gastric mucosa. Also a monoclonal antibody rapid test can be used with gastric washings, feces, and formalin-fixed tissues. PCR is also a highly specific means for identification and specific characterization of *Cryptosporidium* organisms. However, the expense of the equipment, reagents and the trained personnel essential for PCR make this modality most practical in a certified diagnostic clinical laboratory setting. The monoclonal antibody test kits are relatively inexpensive and simple to run in a clinical setting.

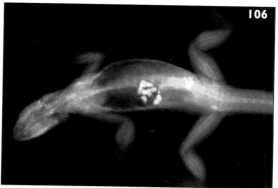

106 i. What is your interpretation/diagnosis of the lizard in Figure 106?
ii. What is the etiology of this condition?
iii. How would you treat this lizard?
iv. What is the prognosis?

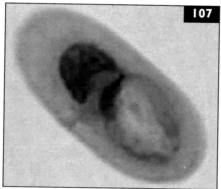

107 i. Identify the organism within the green iguana's (*Iguana iguana*) erythrocyte shown in Figure 107.
ii. Is this organism of pathogenic significance? If so, in what way?

106 i. Nutritional secondary hyperparathyroidism. Note the multilimb long bone periosteal reactions, marked cross-sectional thickening and pathological fractures of long bones. In addition, there are ingested gastrointestinal foreign bodies and intraurocystic calculi.

ii. The most common etiologies for this condition are:
- Hypocalcemia.
- Hyperphosphatemia.
- Hypovitaminosis D-3.
- Renal insufficiency permitting the loss of calcium and the retention of phosphorus.
- Primary hyperparathyroidsm due to parathyroid hormone-secreting adenomatous parathyroid neoplasms.

NOTE: the ingested foreign bodies are probably stones and should readily pass with the feces of this lizard. The radio-opaque objects within the urinary bladder are sufficiently small to permit them to pass through the urodeum safely – unless they grow larger with time.

iii. Depending upon the etiology, treatment is directed at:
- Re-establishing a normal blood calcium to phosphorus ratio to one with a more natural Ca:P ratio of at least 2:1.
- Increasing blood levels of calcium and reducing blood phosphorus by changing the captive diet to one with adequate calcium and administering exogenous calcium gluconate or calcium lactate orally and/or parenterally; correcting hypovitaminosis D-3 by administration of oral vitamin D-3 and providing UV irradiation by an appropriate natural or artificial exposure to sunlight or a UV-emitting light source, emitting UVB at 280–335 nm. In severe cases, intranasal administration of calcitonin salmon is helpful, but rather expensive.
- Treating any concurrent renal disease.
- Excising a parathyroid adenomatous tumor.

iv. The prognosis is favorable if the patient is treated before hypocalcemia reaches a fatally low level where cardiac muscle function, nerve conduction and/or blood coagulation are impeded.

107 i. *Schellackia iguanae.*
ii. *Schellackia* is not of pathogenic significance under most circumstances. Often it is an incidental finding during routine microscopic examination of stained blood films from *wild-caught* iguanas. If it is identified in a captive iguana, it is highly likely that the lizard was *not* captive bred and, thus, it is of potential use in forensic investigations of an animal's origin claimed as being from a captive bred provenance.

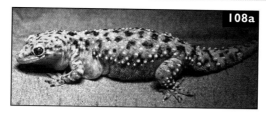

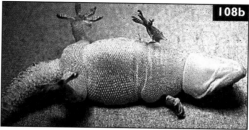

108 The gecko shown in Figures **108a, 108b** had a history of progressive lethargy, anorexia, massive coelomic distention and subcutaneous edema.

i. What is your interpretation of this leopard gecko's (*Eublepharis macularius*) medical condition? Specifically, what organ systems could be malfunctioning or insufficiently functioning?

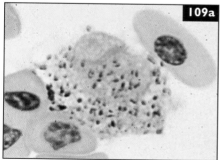

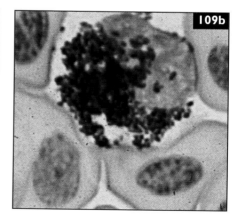

109 What is the nature of the intracytoplasmic objects contained in the two cells illustrated in Figure **109a, 109b**?

108 i. The organ systems that *could* be involved in this gecko's medical condition include any or all of the following potential dysfunctions/abnormalities:
• Myocardial insufficiency.
• Renal insufficiency.
• Hepatic insufficiency.
• Intestinal, via a protein-wasting enteropathy.
• Nutritional: hypoproteinemia (possible but unlikely in this instance).

NOTE: in this instance, a full necropsy and histopathological examination revealed the following significant abnormalities:
• Extensive hepatic fibrosis.
• Diffuse renal interstitial fibrosis.
• Intestinal coccidiosis; thus an etiology for a protein-wasting enteropathy.
• Peribulbar abscessation; this lesion likely did NOT contribute to the intracoelomic ascites nor the subcutaneous edema.

109 Engulfed (phagocytized) bacteria.

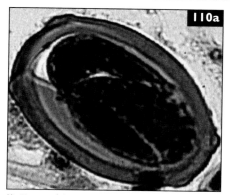

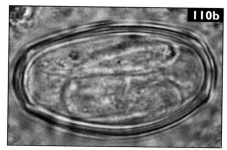

110 i. Identify these two parasitic ova from the feces of monitor (varanid) lizards (**110a, 110b**).

ii. Does this parasite employ an indirect or direct life cycle?

111 Identify this popular amphibian 'pet' (**111**).

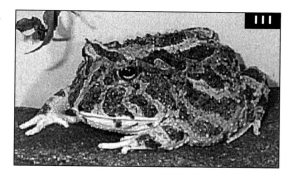

112 Figure **112a** shows the glass front of a cage in a European reptile collection. Note the abraded glass near the bottom of the panel caused by the frequent pacing by one or more of the cage's inhabitants.

i. What can you suggest that would lessen this incessant stereotypical behavior?

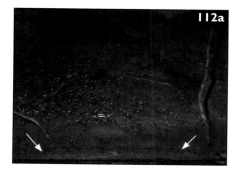

110 i. Embryonated *Spiruroid* ova.
ii. A direct life cycle.

111 Argentine horned frog, (*Ceratophrys ornate*) also known as the 'Pac Man' frog. Note: there are several color morphs of this frog available in the pet trade. Shown is the natural coloration and pattern of this frog.

112 i. Pacing and other stereotypical behavior often can be lessened by the addition of an opaque visual barrier to the captive environment (**112b**).
NOTE: the addition of cage 'furniture' such as rocks, hollow logs, trees and/or branches, water containers in which the animals can soak, etc. also enhances the captive environment and lessens stereotypical repetitive behaviors. Such additions also improve the viewing experience of those who visit such exhibits.

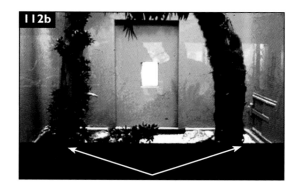

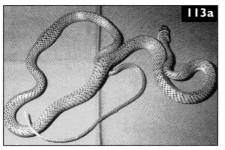
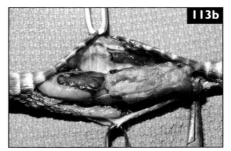

113 i. What are some tentative diagnostic possibilities for this tropical rat snake's (*Elaphe* sp.) medical condition (**113a, 113b**)?
ii. What tests or diagnostic procedures would you perform to aid in confirming your diagnosis?

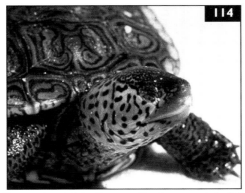

114 What is your diagnosis of this diamondback terrapin's (*Malaclemys terrapin*) appearance (**114**)?

113 i. Tentative diagnoses include all of the following possibilities for this snake's intracoelomic swelling:
- Inflammatory mass: abscess, pyogranuloma.
- Cystic space-occupying lesion: endocrine, renal, parasitic or inclusion cyst; obstructed ureter; products of conception: abnormal or mummified egg, etc.
- Neoplastic mass: adenoma, squamous cell carcinoma, adenocarcinoma, lymphoreticular tumor, neural cell tumor, sarcoma.
- Foreign body reaction.
- Vascular anomaly, aneurysm.

ii. Diagnostic procedures include:
- Radiography.
- Ultrasonography: Doppler blood flow detection.
- Fine-needle aspirate biopsy (with or without image guidance).
- Celioscopy.
- Open (celiotomy) biopsy.

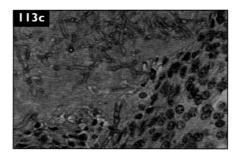

The confirmed diagnosis was mycotic nephritis. Figure **113c** shows a fungal-stained (PAS × 240 original modification) histological section of the mass that effaced much of the snake's kidney.

Note the numerous red-staining, septated fungal mycelia.

114 Anophthalmia. Note the total absence of the right eye; this anomaly was bilateral. Both microphthalmia and anophthalmia are relatively common developmental defects encountered in chelonians and snakes. In some chelonian neonates, anophthalmia, as well as several other anomalies, has been traced to abnormally elevated incubation temperatures during the early stages of embryonic development.

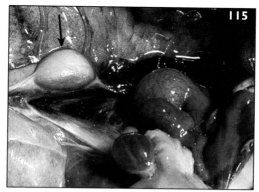

115 Identify the organ at the end of the black arrow in Figure **115**, an interoperative photographic image of surgery in a green iguana (*Iguana iguana*); the head is to the right.

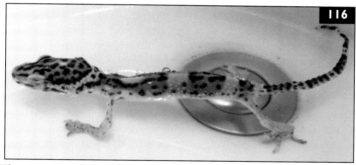

116 i. What is your diagnosis/interpretation of the leopard gecko (*Eublepharis macularius*) soaking in a basin of water in Figure **116**?
ii. Given its emaciated appearance, how would you treat it (1) immediately and, (2) during the next 2 weeks (assuming that it lived that long)?
iii. What is the prognosis?

115 Right testis.

116 i. Severe inanition. Leopard geckos are characterized by their well fleshed, even 'chubby' tails in which they store energy-rich fat. Note the whispy tail that appears devoid of any fatty or even discernable skeletal muscle tissue. Furthermore, its limbs appear to have lost most of their skeletal muscle tissue. In addition, there is signficant retained periocular skin adhering to the eyelids. Without appropriate food, the body first calls upon stored fat as an energy resource. When the adipose tissue is exhausted, the next tissue to be sacrificed is skeletal muscle protein. The very last resources are the liver and brain.

ii. This lizard has little, if any, energy resource(s) upon which to call in times of any stress. Therefore, it is essential to handle it with great care to avoid any further trauma or excessive stress. This is particularly germane during the initial treatment. It should be rehydrated with physiological fluid(s) containing both electrolytes, as well as an immediate energy source in the form of soluble carbohydrate and, if possible, protein hydrolysate such as casein powder diluted with water. Once the gecko has been properly rehydrated, and appears to be resuscitated sufficiently, it can be hand-fed or tube-fed *very* gently – and, using *minimal physical restraint* – with a readily digested and assimilated food source such as small amounts of diluted fruit nectar, cane sugar syrup and supplemented with modest amounts of vitamin–mineral powder, tofu bean cake and/or beaten raw egg. These may be added to the slurry-like gruel being fed via pipette or stomach tube. If necessary, it can be introduced via the esophagus with a small-bore pliable feeding tube or soft rubber urinary catheter. It is essential that all of these treatments are administered with the utmost gentleness. The administration of adrenal corticosteroids and prophylactic antibiotics in the absence of evident infection and in such a severely labile patient is controversial and should be decided on a case-by-case basis.

iii. The prognosis is guarded because of the severity of the chronic starvation/inanition/dehydration that was evident when the gecko was first presented. Moreover, the likelihood that the catabolism of skeletal muscle as an energy source, in the absence of adequate hydration (and, thus, renal perfusion), may have *already* induced excessive accumulation of urates within this gecko's renal glomerular filtration and tubular excretory system, resulting in visceral gout and significant renal insufficiency. Certainly, attempts at compassionate resuscitation are worthy of the effort, but so much damage may already have been occurred, that all measures may fail – as they did in this instance.

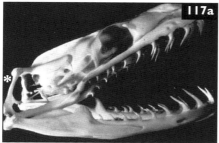

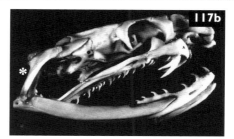

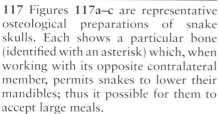

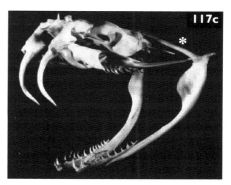

117 Figures **117a–c** are representative osteological preparations of snake skulls. Each shows a particular bone (identified with an asterisk) which, when working with its opposite contralateral member, permits snakes to lower their mandibles; thus it possible for them to accept large meals.

i. What is the name of this pair of bones:
A, sphenoid;
B, quadrate;
C, innominate;
D, malleus?

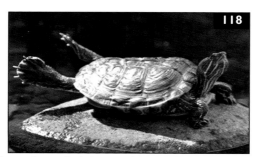

118 i. What is the red-eared slider turtle (*Trachemys scripta elegans*) doing in Figure **118**?
ii. What is the purpose for this behavior?

117 i. B, quadrate bones. Working in concert with its opposite number and the mandibles, which are not fused securely together at the mandibular symphysis, some snakes can swallow enormous meals that would appear, at first glance, to be physically impossible.

118 i. Basking; thermoregulating.
ii. Increasing its internal, deep core, temperature by exposing itself maximally to solar (or, when indoors, exposed to artificial sources of external artificial illumination) warmth. Once the turtle's deep core temperature is sufficiently warmed, it will usually return to the water or shade so as not to overheat.

119 i. Identify the object protruding from this chameleon's cloacal vent (**119a, 119b**).
ii. How do you explain its presence behind the lizard?
iii. How would you treat this patient?
iv. What is your prognosis?

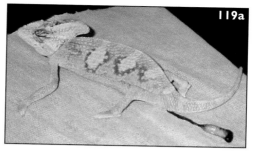

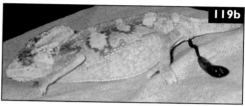

120 Identify this popular 'pet' lizard (**120**).

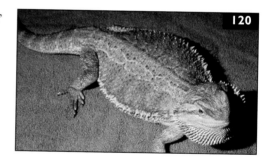

121 Figure **121** was recorded whilst performing a necropsy on a South American boa constrictor (*Boa c. constrictor*).
i. Identify the multiple pale lesions exhibited in these five liver slices.
ii. What is the organism that induces this characteristic lesion?

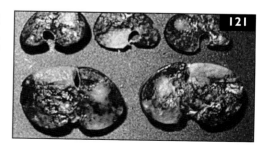

119 i. The object is the chameleon's tongue.

ii. The only explanation possible is that the animal swallowed his tongue and passed it through his digestive tract.

iii. The tongue must be amputated.

iv. The prognosis, surprisingly, is favorable for a *captive* chameleon, because these lizards soon learn to take prey offered to them with forceps. In the wild, a chameleon lacking its tongue would likely be unable to seize and swallow its usual agile and winged insect prey.

120 Australasian bearded dragon lizard (*Pogona vitticeps*).

121 i. Multifocal hepatic infarcts.

ii. The protozoan parasite, *Entamoeba invadens*.

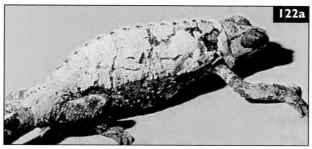

122 What is your interpretation of this lizard's integumentary condition (**122a**)?

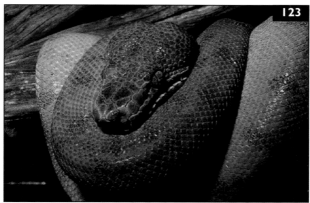

123 Identify the snake in Figure **123**.

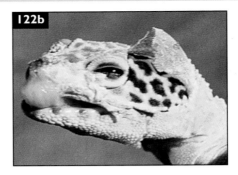

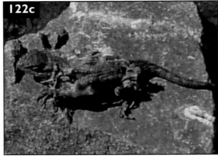

122 Ecdysis. Although this chameleon is shedding its old epidermis in a piecemeal fashion, it is a normal behavior for some lizards, especially some species of chameleons, geckos and small iguanids (**122b, 122c**).

123 Emerald tree boa, *Corallus caninus*.

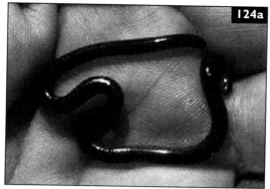

124 i. This is the smallest snake in the world. Identify the tiny snake (**124a**).
ii. What do these snakes eat?
iii. What feature of its reproductive behavior is so interesting and highly unusual?

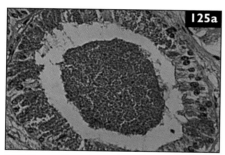 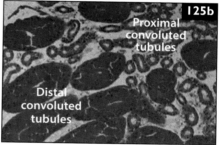

125 Some lizards and snakes possess a modification of their renal distal convoluted tubules, known as the *sexual segment*. Tall columnar epithelial cells lining the tubules are hypertrophied and secrete a distinctly granular material into the lumen of these modified tubules (**125a, 125b**).
i. What is the function of this granular secretion?
ii. Is it present in both genders? If not, in which gender is it found?

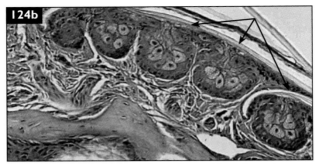

124 i. It is a so-called 'worm' snake, *Rhamphotyphlops barmina*.

ii. The diet of these small snakes consists of tiny invertebrates.

iii. These snakes are parthenogenetic and, thus, uniparental. They consist of only females which give birth to daughters that are essentially genetic clones of their mothers and grandmothers.

AUTHOR'S NOTE: interestingly, these diminutive snakes are burrowing creatures, that do possess eyes but, because they spend most of their time beneath the surface of the soil in which they live, they must rely upon their tongue and specialized sense organs located beneath the epidermis of their rostrums to sense and locate their tiny insect prey. Figure **124b** is a photomicrograph of a thin microsection that illustrates several of these touch corpuscle-like sensory structures (arrows).

125 i. H&E-stained histological sections of a lizard's (**125a**) and snake's (**125b**) renal distal convoluted tubule showing the typical sexual segment granular material being secreted by the tubule's epithelial cells into the lumen of the tubule. It is believed that this secretion possesses a pheromone-like function that influences territoriality and sexual behavior.

ii. It is characteristic in the *male* gender of the reptiles in which it is known to exist. When identified, the sexual segment can be used to determine the gender of the lizard or snake from whose kidney tissue it was found. Thus it can be a useful clue in forensic cases in which the gender of the animal was not known beforehand.

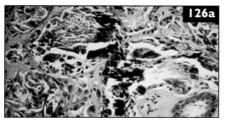

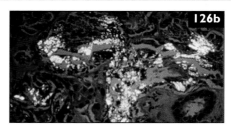

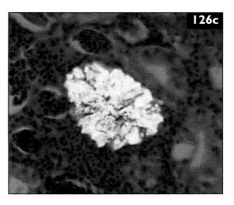

126 Figures **126a**, **126b** are paired images of photomicroscopic stained kidney sections with plain, and then cross-polarized illumination. Figure **126c** was made with solely cross-polarized illumination.
i. What is the nature of the brightly refracted material revealed in the cross-polarized photomicrographs?

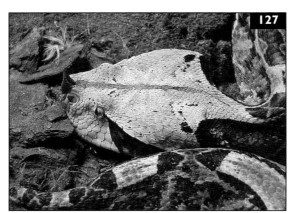

127 A client comes to your clinic with the following animal (**127**). Before examining it and treating it, it is helpful to identify it.
i. What is your identification of this snake?

126 Cholesterol crystal deposits within the renal tissues. These crystals are most often identified in reptiles fed canned dog or cat food.

127 i. It is a rhinoceros viper (*Bitis nasicornis*), a very close cousin to a Gaboon viper (*Bitis gabonica*). Thus, if you are going to handle this snake, exercise great caution to avoid being bitten and envenomated! They possess elongated fangs and potent venom.

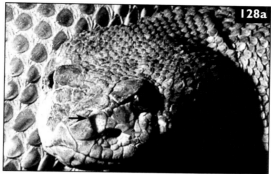

128 Figure **128a** of a North American rattlesnake (*Crotalus* sp.) shows the left respiratory nare and left facial pit organ (back and red arrows, respectively).
i. What is the function of the paired facial pit organs?

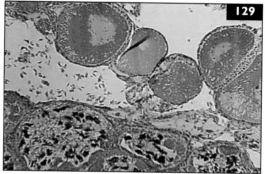

129 While performing a microscopic examination of stained histopathological sections from a North American western toad, you observe the field shown in Figure **129**.
i. How do you explain the observation of *both* typical ovarian tissue with characteristic follicular development, as well as well as typical testicular tissue with maturing spermatozoa? Is it: A, evidence of *true* hermaphroditism; B, evidence of a *pseudo*hermaphroditism; C, Bidder's organ; D, an artefact of histological processing?

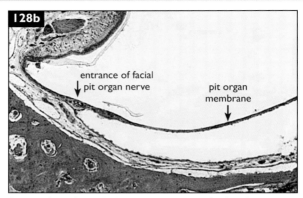

Figure 128b shows a histological photomicrograph of a facial pit organ sensory membrane.

128 i. The facial pit organs are exquisitely sensitive to differences in thermal signals they receive from the environment and are employed in prey perception and following, as well as detection of potential predators or other animals to which the snake may be exposed and injured.

129 i. C, Bidder's organ, an entirely normal structure and present as a 'cap' at one pole of the ovary. It is a characteristic of some North American species of toads of the species *Bufo*.

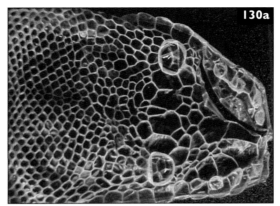

130 Figure **130a** shows a portion of the recently shed epidermis of a ball (or regal) python (*Python regius*) and the head of the snake itself.
i. What is your interpretation/diagnosis of this snake's tertiary spectacle shield?
ii. What is the likely etiology of this condition?

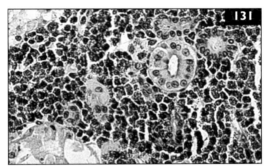

131 i. Identify the myriad number of small cells with orange-red intracytoplasmic granules infiltrating the tissues comprising the interstitial tissues in this snake's kidney (**131**).
ii. What is the significance of these cells?

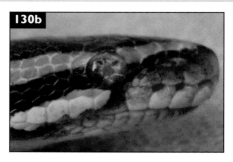

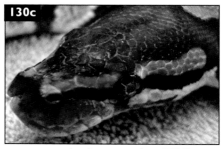

130 i. Variant scale pattern on both spectacles. While most ball pythons have spectacles that are smooth as observed in other snakes, others of this taxon are occasionally observed with this anomaly. Figures **130b, 130c** show both eyes of this snake prior to its most recent ecdysis.
ii. This anomaly was most likely the result of a point mutation in this snake.

131 i. The cells are heterophil granulocytes.
ii. These cells are the reptilian counterpart of mammalian neutrophils and are commonly observed in sites of infection, especially of bacterial etiology. In this instance, the diagnosis was suppurative interstitial nephritis.

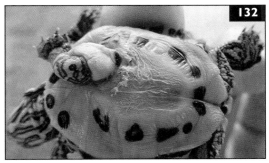

132 What is the proper terminology to describe the anomaly exhibited by the juvenile turtle shown in Figure **132**?

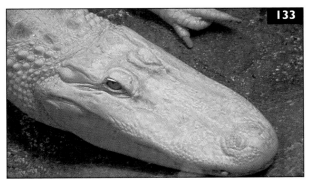

133 How would you describe this American alligator's (*Allilgator mississippiensis*) color (**133**)?
i. Which of the following best answers this question: A, albinism; B, hypoerythritism; C, hypoxanthism; D, hypomelanism?

132 Limb duplication; supernumerary fifth limb.

133 i. D, hypomelanism. This animal is *not* a true albino. True albinistic animals lack colored pigments in their chromatophores and, as a result, appear white or pale pink and usually possess pink or red iridies. Hypomelanistic animals are deficient in the amount of brown or black melanin pigment contained in their epidermal chromatophores (melanophores), but may exhibit relatively normal melanin pigmentation in their irides. Hypoerythristic animals lack or have reduced red pigment(s) in their epidermal erythrophores. Hypoxanthistic animals lack yellow pigment(s) within their xanthophores.

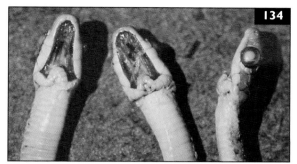

134 Figure **134** shows three neonate garter snakes, (*Thamnophis s. sirtalis*), each of which displays a severe developmental anomaly.
i. What is the term for this?

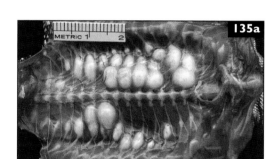

135 Figure **135a** shows the opened body of a juvenile monitor lizard (*Varanus* sp.).
i. What is your interpretation/diagnosis of this young lizard's condition that is affecting its ribs?
ii. Which of the following best describes the etiology of this condition: A, inflammatory/infectious; B, neoplastic; C, aberrant skeletal growth?

134 i. Mandibular agenesis, agnathism. Whether this case of multiple siblings being affected with the same developmental anomaly is genetic (heritable) or epigenetic (not necessarily heritable, but due to some environmental cause) is not known. For instance, when some tortoise and crocodilian eggs are incubated at abnormally high, yet sub-lethal, temperatures they are known to result in deformed neonates with a variety of developmental anatomical anomalies.

135 i. Osteochondroma (osteocartilaginous exostoses).
ii. B, neoplastic etiology (**135b**).

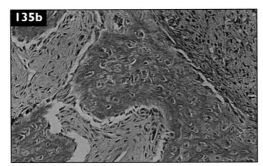

135b Histological section of one of the osteocartilagenous exostoses. Note the aberrant growth of partially mineralized cartilaginous tissue and the intervening spaces filled with fibrocollagenous tissue.

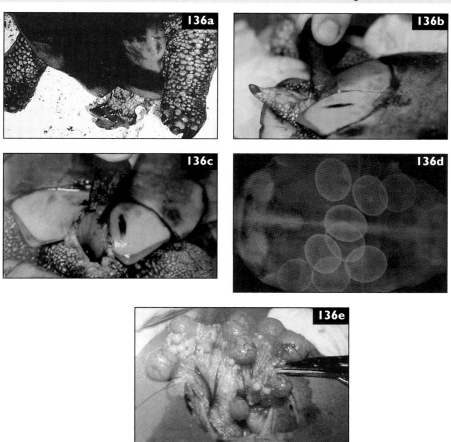

136 Figures **136a–e** show an adult Hermann's tortoise (*Testudo hermanni*).
i. How do you reconcile this adult tortoise which possesses the external physical characteristics and an erectile penis, with the presence of what appear to be normal shelled ova within its oviducts? Is the answer: A, the tortoise is a true hermaphrodite; B, the tortoise is a pseudohermaphrodite?

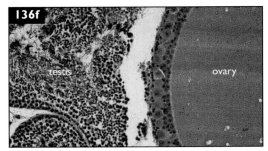

136 i. B, a pseudohermaphrodite.

NOTE: during exploratory celiotomy, this tortoise was found to have numerous developing ova and early follicular development; however, no testes were identified. Therefore, the tortoise was a *pseudo*hermaphrodite, possessing fully functioning ovaries and a penis-like phallus, but no testes. Whether the phallus was an actual penis or a hypertrophied clitoris is unclear; however, its histological characteristics were consistent with those of a true penis.

For reference purposes, Figure **136f** is a photomicrograph of a North American fence or 'swift' lizard (*Sceloporus* sp.), that was a *true* hermaphrodite. Note the separate and distinct ovarian and testicular tissues present. Interestingly, these tissues were separate and not conjoined in an ovotestis as is often found in many other true hermaphroditic animals. Also, why androgenic and estrogenic hormones failed to inhibit their opposite gender's development is unknown.

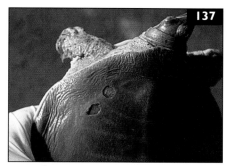

137 Soft-shell turtles, *Apalone* sp. are particularly prone to develop ulcerative dermal lesions on both their pliable and delicate carapace and plastron, as well as on the integument of their extremities (137).
i. What is the most common microorganism cultured from these lesions?

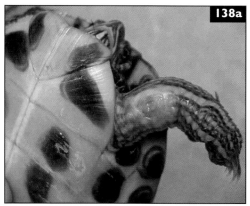

138 The juvenile semi-aquatic turtle shown in Figure 138a has a swollen and discolored left fore-limb.
i. What is your provisional diagnosis?
ii. What diagnostic procedures would you employ to confirm your diagnosis?
iii. How would you treat this patient?

137 i. *Citrobacter freundii*. The condition is termed SCUD and is highly contagious to tank-mates and also to humans not wearing protective gloves.

138 i. The lesion is most likely an abscess or pyogranuloma.
ii. After appropriate sedation and anesthesia, the altered skin overlying the swelling is incised and the contents of the lesion are evacuated. The inspissated contents of the abscess cavity should be subjected to microbioloigcal culture and antibiotic sensitivity testing to ascertain the most effective antibiotic to administer for this infection.
iii. The cavity is flushed with 0.75% chlorhexidine diacetate (or gluconate) solution or dilute povidone iodine solution, and, if appropriate, packed with gauze soaked in the same disinfectant that was used for flushing the abscess cavity. A parenteral antibiotic is administered and supportive nursing that includes fluid therapy is given, to ensure adequate renal perfusion. The turtle should be kept dry until the lesion heals from the inside outward. If necessary, the infected site can be temporarily covered with a liquid plastic bandage to permit the animal to feed normally in clean water once or twice weekly. An image of the evacuated abscess and its contents is shown in Figure 138b.

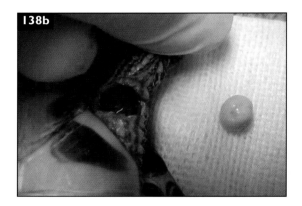

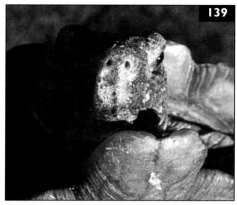

139 What is your interpretation/diagnosis of the tortoise illustrated in Figure 139?

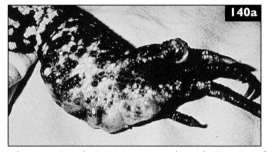

140a Figure 140a shows a South American tegu lizard (*Tupinambis teguixin*) with a swollen left hind-foot. Note the multiple soft fluctuant swellings.
i. What is your provisional diagnosis of this lizard's condition?
ii. What tests or procedures would you perform to confirm your diagnosis?
iii. How would you treat or manage this patient?
iv. What is your prognosis?

139 Chronic respiratory infection. This condition can be the result of a viral infection, especially chelonian herpesvirus and/or *Mycoplasma* infections, as well as a wide variety of bacterial pathogens or a combination of more than a single pathogen.

140 i. The most likely provisional diagnosis is an infection.

ii. Appropriate tests are:

- Obtain one or more specimens of exudate for microbiological culture and antibiotic sensitivity testing.
- A cytological examination of the exudate might also be helpful.
- A radiograph of the affected foot would provide an estimate of any osseous involvement secondary to the infectious process.

iii. Depending upon the results of the tests above, the affected foot can be opened aseptically for thorough incision and drainage of the multiple lesions. If radiography revealed extensive osteolysis, or if the incision and drainage disclosed widespread infection so severe as to confirm that spread of infective secondary foci to distant organs, amputation of the entire limb via a coxofemoral disarticulation would be preferable.

The microbiological culture and sensitivity testing disclosed infection by *Dermatophilus congolensis*. The tegu lizard was anesthetized and the entire left hind-limb was prepared for aseptic surgery.

Figure **140b** shows the incised limb. Note the multiple abscesses surrounded by dense fibrous capsules (black arrows). This encapsulation of the abscesses would very likely have impeded effective penetration of any antibiotic agent. Because of this fact and also the multifocal distribution of these inflammatory lesions, as well as the zoonotic public health significance of the etiological infective agent, the entire left hind-limb was amputated at the coxofemoral articulation, thus, leaving no stump to be abraded or otherwise traumatized. The lizard was continued on the antibiotic shown to be most effective during culture and antibiotic sensitivity testing.

iv. The tegu made an uneventful recovery and had no recurrence of inflammatory lesions during the next 2 years of observation.

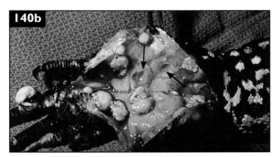

140b Surgical specimen of the tegu lizard's left foot. Note the multiple abscesses surrounded by thick and dense fibrous capsules (arrows) that made this case so challenging.

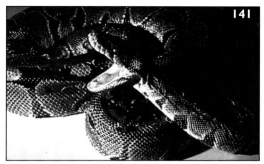

141 What is your interpretation of this ball or regal python's (*Python regius*) condition (**141**)?

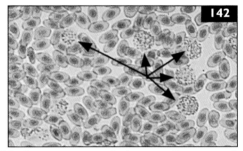

142 In Figure **142** black arrows are pointing to cells scattered throughout this stained blood film.
i. Identify these cells.
ii. What does the relative number of these cells signify or strongly suggest?

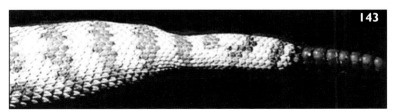

143 **i.** What is the gender of this North American rattlesnake (*Crotalus* sp.) (**143**)?
ii. On what criterion did you base your answer?

141 The python is exhibiting open-mouth breathing which can signify any of the following possible disease conditions:
- A respiratory condition, either upper or lower in location.
- A bacterial, fungal, or viral pneumonia.
- A metazoan parasitic infestation with a lungworm or lung fluke.
- Dyspnea related to the covering of one or both external nares by unshed epidermal remnants. Note the unshed epidermis on this snake's body.
- The accumulation of inspissated mucus covering and/or within the upper respiratory system.
- Tracheal chondromata which are relatively common in ball pythons.
- The aforementioned dysecdysis.

142 i. Heterophil granulocytes. These are the reptilian equivalent to and comparable in function with mammalian neutrophils.
ii. When increased in number, heterophilia suggests a bacterial infection.

143 i. It is a female.
ii. In males, the paired hemipenes impart a much fuller, more gradually tapering appearance to the postcloacal tail shape.

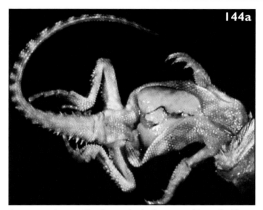

144 Figure **144a** shows a juvenile bearded dragon lizard, *Pogona henrylawsoni*, with its body cavity opened during a necropsy examination.
i. Identify the major abnormality shown.

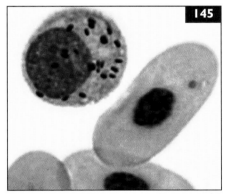

145 Identify the cell in the center of this image of a stained blood film (**145**).

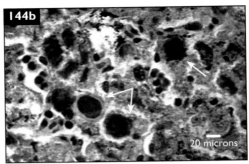

144b Photomicrograph of liver section from this lizard. Note the large intranuclear inclusion bodies (white arrows).

144 i. The liver is swollen and an abnormally pale tan color. Figure **144b** is a photomicrograph of a histological section made from this lizard's liver. Note the densely staining viral inclusion bodies. These enormous inclusion bodies were characterized by electron microscopy as an adenovirus.

145 A lymphocyte with engulfed bacteria and cellular debris.

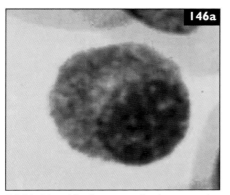
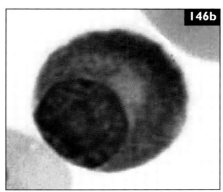

146 i. Identify these two leukocytes shown in Figures **146a, 146b**.
ii. What does an abnormally large number of these cells suggest?

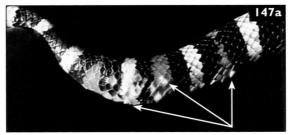

147 Figure **147a** shows a milk snake (*Lampropeltis triangulum*) with a diffuse dermatopathy consisting of many scales being elevated and displaying a white base to each affected scale. This condition had been present for over 1 month.
i. What are the major consequences of ignoring this type of ailment and permitting it to go untreated?

146 i. These cells are plasmacytes. Note their eccentric nuclei, dark bluish cytoplasm and clear perinuclear halo.
ii. Increased numbers of these cells suggest an immune reaction; vastly increased numbers may signify multiple myeloma, a plasmacytic lymphoreticular neoplasm.

147 i. The snake has a suppurative dermatitis. Left untreated, an infection such as this can gain entry into the vascular system and become widely disseminated. Figure **147b** shows the snake's liver. Note the leukocytic infiltrate comprising this focus of hepatitis and the vacuolar hepatocellular lipidosis, which was incidental to the inflammatory reaction. Similar inflammatory infiltrates were identified throughout this snake's visceral organs.

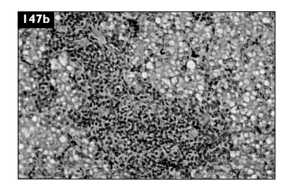

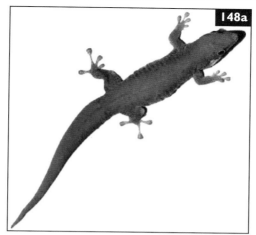

148 Figure **148a** is of a gecko, *Phelsuma grandis*, on a clean glass surface. Many species of geckos can move comfortably over ultra-smooth perpendicular glass surfaces. Some of these lizards are also able to run when fully inverted (upside down) on smooth surfaced ceilings.
i. How do these lizards accomplish these feats?

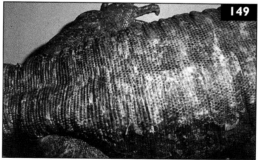

149 Figure **149** shows a red tegu lizard (*Tupinambis rufescens*) with a dermatopathy consisting of severe hyperkeratosis to the point of significant skin thickening.
i. What dietary deficiency is most likely to induce this integumentary alteration?
ii. Given that this lizard was a long-term captive 'pet' reptile, what do you think induced this dietary deficiency?
iii. How would you treat this condition and prevent it in the future?

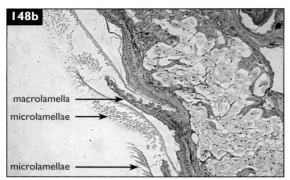

148b Photomicrograph of a seta from the ventral toepad of a gecko illustrating the macrolamellae and microlamellae with which geckos grip even glass-smooth surfaces.

148 i. The toe pads of these lizards are covered with setae composed of macrolamellae, which are further divided into myriad numbers of microlamellae. It is with these structures that enable the lizards' feet to grip tiny irregularities on the surfaces upon which they walk – even when suspended upside-down (**148b**).

149 i. Hypovitaminosis A.
ii. In captivity, these lizards are most often fed a diet of small rodents, which may or may not have gut contents with sufficient preformed vitamin A. However, in their wild state, these lizards consume a diet of small mammals, birds, reptiles, invertebrates, as well as scavenged ripe fallen fruit from a variety of tropical fruit trees, especially figs and mangoes. A high protein diet, lacking in either preformed vitamin A, or carotenoids from which they can synthesize their own vitamin A, can result in a vitamin A deficiency with its attendant induction of hyperkeratosis.
iii. The addition of orange and yellow vegetables such as cooked squash, carrots, and colorful orange and yellow fruits to the diet of these usually carnivorous lizards will usually treat and prevent this dermatopathy from occurring. In severe cases, an initial *oral* administration of preformed vitamin A can be administered.

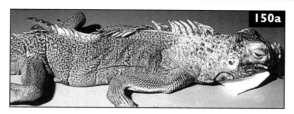

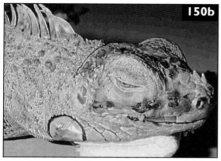
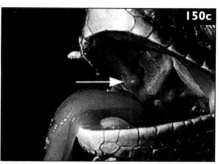

150 Figures 150a–c depict a profoundly depressed juvenile green iguana (*Iguana iguana*). The lizard is underweight and exhibits multifocal inflammatory lesions on its head. During a physical examination of this lizard, multiple pale raised lesions are found immediately subjacent to the oral mucosal epithelium (150c).
i. Considering the general appearance and lethargy displayed by this iguana, what is your tentative diagnosis?
ii. What specific tests or procedures would confirm your diagnostic impression?
iii. What is the prognosis discussed with this iguana's owner *before* discussing the treatment for this iguana's medical problem? Why?
The relevant hematology results were as follows:

RBC	960,000/mm^3 (960 × 10^9/l)
WBC	24,300/mm^3 (24.3 × 10^9/l)
Heterophils	79%
Lymphocytes	4%
Monocytes	11%
Azurophils	6%
Basophils	0%
Eosinophils	0%
Thrombocytes	Slightly diminished

150 i. This iguana's multiple cutaneous inflammatory lesions, together with the oral foci are highly suggestive of the hematogenous dissemination of pathogenic microorganisms. Judging from the poor condition exhibited by this iguana and the history provided by its owner, its current disease was not particularly acute; it had not been eating for at least several weeks, perhaps longer. Thus, this patient may have been developing this condition for many weeks. Once the pathogenic bacteria gained entrance to the vascular system, infective microemboli could have readily spread to vitally important visceral organs.

ii. The hemogram revealed that there was a significant leukocytosis, heterophilia and lymphopenia. The monocytes were slightly above normal, which suggests that the infection is chronic, rather than acute.

iii. Appropriate diagnostic tests include microbiological culture and antibiotic sensitivity testing, hematologic examination of whole blood and a complete blood count, blood microbiological culture and sensitivity testing, cytological examination of exudate specimens, and, especially, Doppler blood flow ultrasonography of the heart and its valves and outflow tract vessels. This technology is helpful in assessing

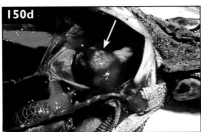

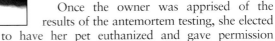

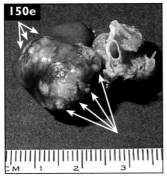

whether the infection in this lizard extended far beyond the obvious integumentary and oral tissues and had seeded the heart valves. Where economic constraints limit the choices of diagnostic procedures, a Doppler blood flow study often can detect significant extraneous blood flow sounds. It is noninvasive and relatively inexpensive.

Once the owner was apprised of the results of the antemortem testing, she elected to have her pet euthanized and gave permission for a full necropsy (150d–f). Note the extensive pyogranulomatous inflammation of the myocardium.

Note the infiltration and replacement of the myocardium with caseous exudates. Doppler ultrasonic blood flow studies of this lizard revealed extremely abnormal cardiovascular sounds. The origin of these sounds was confirmed to be the distorted heart valve leaflets and their supportive myocardial basal tissues. A significant amount of myocardial tissue had been replaced with pyogranulomatous tissue; thus it was astonishing that the heart could function as an effective pump.

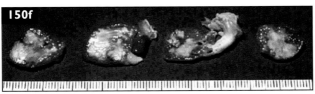

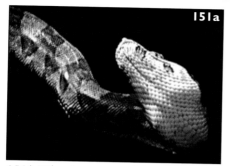

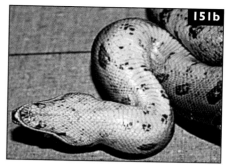

151 i. What is your provisional diagnosis of a snake exhibiting the clinical sign(s) shown by the three different boa constrictors in Figures 151a–c?
ii. What are some etiologies for this clinical manifestation?

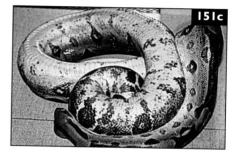

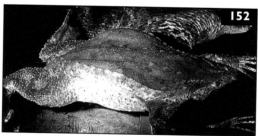

152 Identify this obligatory aquatic amphibian (152).

151 i. The signs displayed are consistent with meningoencephalitis.

ii. The major etiologies for inducing these signs are as follows:
- A bacterial, fungal or viral infection involving the CNS.
- A protozoan, or metazoan parasitism involving the CNS.
- Less common etiologies that could induce similar clinical signs include:
    o A space-occupying lesion involving the CNS.
    o A cyst involving a discrete motor center.
    o A neoplasm, either benign or malignant.
    o A chemical or metabolic derangement creating CNS dysfunction(s):
        - Hypoxemia, severe anemia, some small molecular size agent that is capable of crossing the blood–brain barrier, etc.
        - A vitamin (especially thiamin), or some other essential vitamin B-complex deficiency inducing neural dysfunction.
        - Severe electrolyte excess or deficiency inducing CNS calcium, sodium, potassium (other ionic channel) dysfunction.

Therefore, one must exercise caution when making a diagnosis on a snake exhibiting abnormal postural behavior, sudden blindness, partial (segmental) paresis or paralysis.

152 Surinam toad (*Pipa pipa*).

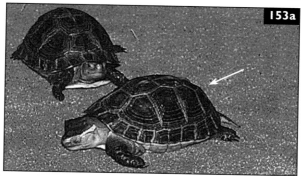

153 i. What is your interpretation of the unanesthetized Asiatic box turtle (*Cuora amboinensis*) shown in the center (white arrow) of Figure **153a**? The other box turtle was normal.

ii. What tests would you employ to confirm your provisional diagnosis?

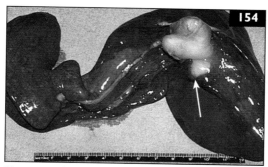

154 Figure **154a** illustrates the liver of an adult California desert tortoise (*Xerobates [Gopherus] agassizi*) recorded during a necropsy.

i. What is your diagnosis?

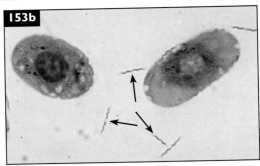

153b Note the spirally coiled spirochete bacteria (arrows).

153 i. The affected turtle appears to be very depressed to the point of being obtunded. Possible etiologies are metabolic disturbances, severe anemia, infections that induce inflammations, intoxications, parasitism, traumatic injuries to the CNS, etc.
ii. Because of the economic concerns involved in clinical diagnostics, particularly when dealing with some reptile-owning clients, this criterion often must be well considered. Three of the least expensive procedures that often yield very important information are:
• A 'multi dip-stick' strip used to test for blood glucose, azotemia, pH, etc.
• A differential blood count, hematocrit (PCV), and thorough microscopic examination of a stained blood film; an automated cell count could miss the presence of non-blood cell constituents.

Figure **153b** reveals the etiology of this turtle's severe depression. The confirmed diagnosis was spirochetemia (black arrows).

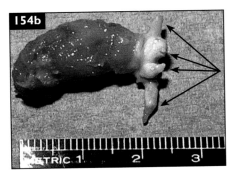

154 i. Chronic suppurative cholecystitis. Figure **154b** shows a cast consisting of inspissated bile, exudates, and cellular debris that faithfully reproduced the major regional biliary tributaries (arrows).

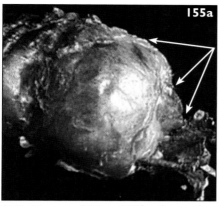 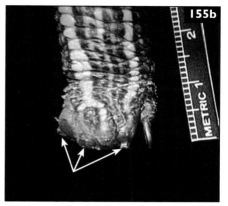

155 Figures **155a, 155b** show the fore-limbs of a red-eared slider turtle (*Trachemys scripta elegans*) whose digits were lost via spontaneous necrosis and autoamputation over a period of approximately 1 year.
i. Based *solely* on this information, what is your tentative diagnosis?
ii. What tests or procedures would you use to confirm your diagnosis?

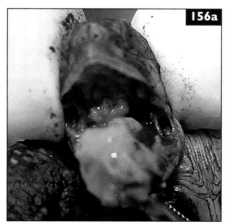

156 Figure **156a** shows a juvenile European tortoise (*Testudo* sp.) with its mouth open revealing abundant thick exudate covering the tongue and palate.
i. What are your tentative diagnoses?
ii. What laboratory tests would you use to help confirm your diagnosis?

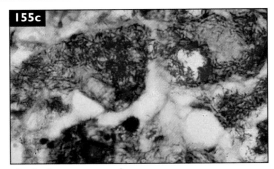

155 i. Mycobacteriosis; lepromatous leprosy.

ii. Cytology, microbiological culture, and histopathology employing special staining, as necessary. In this case, a Fite's modified acid-fast staining revealed myriad numbers of beaded acid-fast microorganisms. Microbiological culture disclosed the organism to be *Mycobacterium ulcerans* (155c). PCR is now routinely performed in many public health laboratories and provides rapid diagnosis.

156 i. This young tortoise exhibits a tenacious exudate adhering to its lingual, palatine and pharyngeal surfaces. The clinical diagnosis is severe exudative glossitis and pharyngitis. The specific diagnosis rests upon characterizing any etiologic agents.

ii. Appropriate examinations include cytology (156b), microbiological culture and antibiotic sensitivity testing and biopsy. When deemed appropriate, viral isolation and/or electron microscopy can be employed to characterize specific viral pathogens accurately.

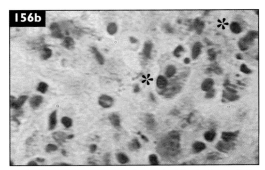

156b Note the large dark-staining intranuclear viral inclusions delineated by black asterisks. The definitive diagnosis was infection with a chelonian herpesvirus.

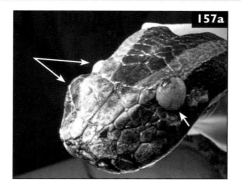

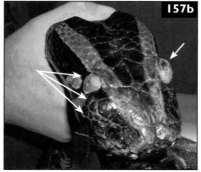

157 Figures **157a, 157b** show a Burmese python (*Python molurus bivittatus*) with a swollen face (white arrows) and bilaterally swollen and opaque tertiary spectacles covering its eyes.

i. What is your diagnosis of this snake's condition?
ii. How would you confirm your diagnosis?
iii. What is your prognosis?
iv. Would you treat this patient? Why?

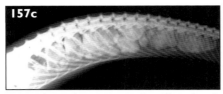

157c

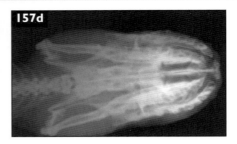

157d

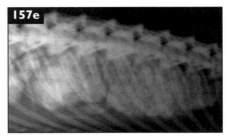

157e

157i. The snake appears to be afflicted with multiple abscesses (pyrogranulomata). The spaces between the tertiary spectacles of both eyes appear to be filled with purulent exudate.

ii. In order to ascertain the extent of the multifocality of these suppurative inflammatory lesions, a complete blood count and whole-body radiography are required (**157c–e**).

One abscess on the right side of the face was incised and drained, leaving a deep cavity (**157f**). Note also the multiple inflammatory foci along the right mandibular dental arcade. The tertiary spectacle is wrinkled and opaque, probably due to its increased thickness and presence of a mass of exudate beneath it.

The radiographs revealed myriad numbers of variably sized round radio-opaque densities scattered throughout the snake's body. These foci are suggestive of widespread dissemination of infection to distant sites, probably via hematogenous distribution of infective microemboli from one abscess to other anatomical locations.

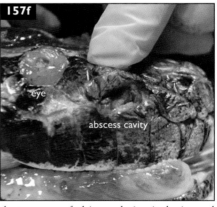

157f

eye

abscess cavity

iii. The prognosis is guarded. It is likely that many of this snake's vital visceral organs are already affected with secondary abscesses arising from the spread from distant sites.

iv. Because of the likely multiplicity of abscesses scattered throughout this snake's body, it is unlikely that it will survive, even after aggressive antibiotic therapy and nursing treatment. Its owner should be appraised of the seriousness of the snake's infection and the likelihood of the necessity for prolonged treatment.

158 i. What is your interpretation of the conditions in which these green turtles (*Chelonia mydas*) are housed (**158**)?
ii. What would you recommend to the owner of these turtles?

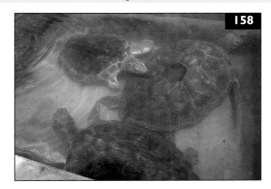

159 What is your diagnosis of this red-eared slider turtle's (*Trachemys scripta elegans*) ophthalmological condition (**159**)?

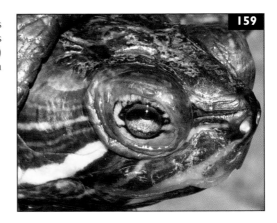

160 i. What is your interpretation/provisional diagnosis of the left fore-limb of the Australasian bearded dragon lizard (*Pogona vitticeps*) shown in Figure **160**?
ii. How would you confirm your diagnosis?
iii. How would you treat or manage this patient?
iv. What is your prognosis?

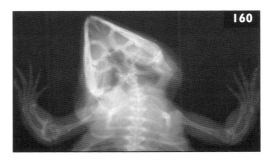

158 i. The turtles are living in overcrowded conditions and the water in which they are confined is turbid and likely contaminated with uneaten food, fecal and urinary wastes. Also, the turtles shown are of significantly different size.
ii. Advice should include reducing animal density, increasing the water flow so as to promote the flushing of wastes, and stocking the tanks with turtles of similar size.

159 Luxated lens.

160 i. The left elbow joint articulation reveals extensive osteolysis and neo-osseous tissue affecting the radial-ulnar-humeral joint. The characteristics of these osteopathies are highly suggestive of an inflammatory process.
ii. A biopsy yielding sufficient material for both microbiological culture and sensitivity, as well as histopathology should narrow the diagnostic possibilities to an infective inflammatory, versus a non-infective autoimmune inflammatory etiology.
iii. If the confirmed etiology is inflammatory due to an infectious process, an intensive course of an appropriate antibiotic may prove effective. If, however, the arthopathy is shown to be an autoimmune process, corticosteroid anti-inflammatory therapy might provide pain relief and return to adequate joint mobility.
iv. The prognosis for return to complete pain-free joint function is guarded. Therefore, an arthrodesis is an option.

161 How would you anesthetize this animal (161)?

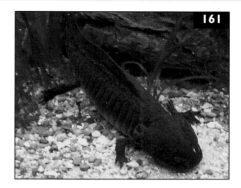

162 What is your diagnosis of the turtle in Figure 162?

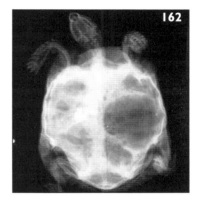

163 What is the gender of this North American semi-aquatic turtle (163a)?

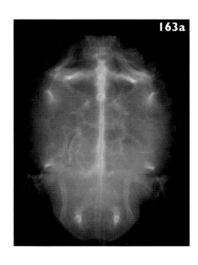

161 Because this axolotl is an aquatic amphibian whose filamentous gills must be kept thoroughly wet in order to function as respiratory gas exchange organs, it is essential to choose a method of anesthesia that permits them to remain submerged. Depending upon what part of the axolotl requires surgical intervention, there are several choices:

1. Regional or local block anesthesia with lidocaine *could* be used for a surgical procedure on a limb or digit; however, it would not be ideal because the animal would be free to move and, thus, pose a problem of restraint.
2. General anesthesia can be accomplished by immersing the animal in a dilute solution of tricaine methanesulfonate (MS222) until a satisfactory level of non-responsiveness is achieved.
3. The axolotl may be placed in a shallow container that permits sufficient water to cover the external gills but not so deep as to cover the entire animal. Then a cotton-tipped applicator is used to distribute or 'paint' alfoxalone acetate/aldolone acetate onto the exposed dorsal integument. This drug is readily absorbed into the skin and achieves surgical anesthesia in only a few minutes. When the surgical procedure is completed, the axolotl should be returned to clean fresh water to recover.

162 Unilateral pneumonia/lung collapse or atelectasis with incomplete aeration of the right lung due to compression from a large gas-filled stomach, which is usually locates to the *left* of the mid-line; in this instance it is seen on the right. The lung-fields of most chelonians occupy the dorsal space from the cranial portion to the caudal portion of the coelomic cavity overlying the pelvic girdle. Incidentally, several radio-opaque objects, probably ingested pebbles, are located left of the stomach and are probably within the lumen of the duodenum.

These objects *could* be obstructing outflow from the stomach.

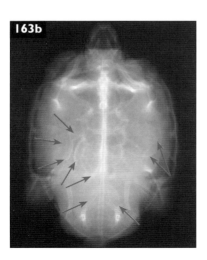

163b

163 Female; there are multiple fractured eggs within the coelom. Figure **163b** shows arrows pointing to numerous fractured/collapsed egg shells.

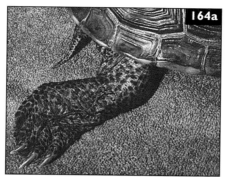

164 Figure **164a** shows the right hind-limb of a North American diamondback terrapin (*Malaclemys terrapin*) whose limb was swollen and was leather-like and firm when palpated. When pinched, the terrapin did not try to withdraw that limb but did actively object when its other three limbs were similarly pressed between thumb and fore-finger. When walking or swimming the terrapin did not use its affected hind-limb. Otherwise, the terrapin ate well and acted normally – except it tended to swim in circles.
i. What are some provisional diagnoses?
ii. What procedures would you perform to help diagnose this animal's condition?

164 i. Possible provisional diagnoses include the following:
- A chronic inflammatory lesion causing the mild swelling, loss of sensation and locomotory function of the affected limb.
- A vascular lesion that gradually involved the blood supply and local nerves that served the affected limb and altered the tissues so that they lost their normal plasticity.
- A lesion induced by the infiltration of neoplastic cells that gradually compressed the nerve supply to the limb.
- A lesion within the vertebral column affecting the spinal cord.
- A focal lesion in the CNS that affected only the right hind-limb. This would be unlikely, but is justified to be placed in the list of possibilities.
- Invasion of the right hind-limb's tissue by a parasitic organism. Again, an unlikely occurrence.

ii. Potentially helpful diagnostic tests or procedures include:
- Radiography.
- Fine-needle aspirate biopsy; followed by: microbiological culture and antibiotic sensitivity testing.
- Doppler ultrasonic blood flow examination to determine adequate blood flow. *At the time that this case was seen, this technology did not exist. Today, it would be one of the first non-invasive tests to be employed.*

Figure **164b** is a radiograph of the affected right hind-limb of the terrapin. Unfortunately, the radiograph did not yield a positive diagnostic clue. Next, a large-bore needle aspiration biopsy was performed under short-term general anesthesia and the cylindrical specimen was divided for culture and sensitivity testing and histopathology (**164c, 164d**).

Based solely upon the histology, the confirmed diagnosis was mycobacteriosis. After 7 weeks of culture, the culture yielded *Mycobacterium chelonei*. Today, PCR testing of specimens can yield accurate results within 24 hours and is available in numerous public health diagnostic laboratories.

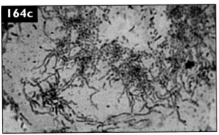

164c Routine cytological stain of exudate aspirated from the terrapin's limb via fine-needle biopsy.

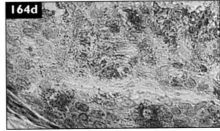

164d Fite's modified acid-fast stain. Note the myriad number of acid-fast microorganisms.

165 i. What is your diagnosis of the chelonian in Figure **165**?
ii. How would you treat this patient for this condition?

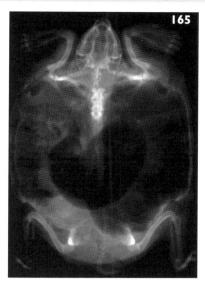

166 Figure **166** is of a green iguana (*Iguana iguana*) with NSHP. What are the characteristic signs of this common nutritional disorder?

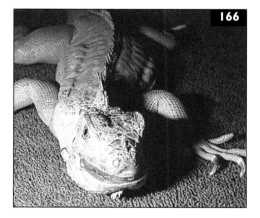

165 i. Gastric dilatation and compression of right lung with mild to moderate atelectasis.

ii. Deflate the gas-filled stomach by either passing a soft feeding tube or fenestrated catheter and/or administer simethicone to break up small gas bubbles to allow the trapped gas to pass. The first of these modalities was employed successfully.

166 This iguana exhibits all of the classic signs of nutritional secondary hyperparathyroidism (NSHP). These are as follows:
- Swollen and deformed mandibles.
- One or more swollen long bones; in this image note the animal's right upper thigh displays this characteristic clinical sign.
- There are rachitic rosettes along the costo-chondral junctions. This is a classical feature of rickets and reflects a failure of the affected bone to mineralize normally, thus creating spherical osteocartilaginous bulges that can be readily seen beneath the skin of the thorax.

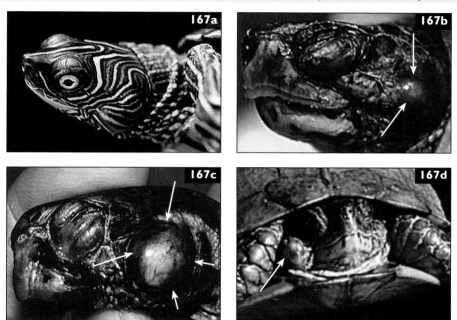

167 Figures 167a–d display lesions (white arrows) that are commonly encountered in both terrestrial and semi-aquatic chelonians.
i. How would you treat this condition?

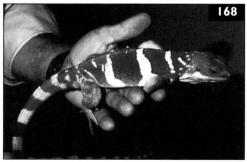

168 i. Identify the reptile in Figure 168.
ii. What is the significance if you see one of these as a patient in private practice?

167 i. These are all abscesses/pyogranulomata and are most effectively treated by incision and drainage, with thorough flushing of the abscess cavity with dilute chlorhexidine diacetate (or gluconate) after the usually solidified purulent exudate has been removed. The abscess cavity is packed with a gauze sponge saturated with the same wound flushing antiseptic solution. If deemed appropriate, a broad-spectrum antibiotic is administered parenterally. Semi-aquatic turtles and terrapins should be kept out of water except for feeding until the skin has covered the site of the abscess. Prior to immersion, the wound sites are covered by a liquid plastic wound dressing.

168 i. This lizard is a Fiji iguana (*Brachylophus faciatus*).
ii. It is an endangered CITES-listed species and, as such, would not normally be in private hands.

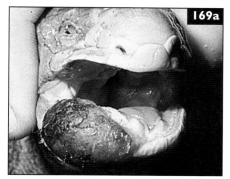

169 The skink in Figure **169a** has a large crusted lesion on its right mandible.
i. What is your diagnosis?
ii. What tests or procedures would your employ immediately to differentiate alternative diagnoses?
iii. How would you treat this patient?
iv. What is the prognosis?

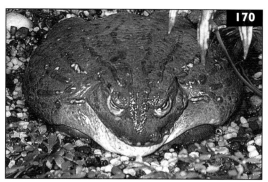

170 What precautions should you observe when handling a patient such as in Figure **170**, and why?

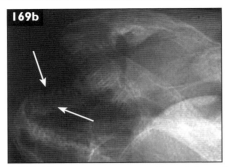

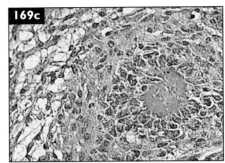

169 i. The mass appears at first sight to be an abscess or pyogranuloma. However, it could also be a neoplasm or parasite-induced inflammatory granuloma. There is a possibility that the underlying mandible could be involved.

ii. Radiography is non-invasive and would reveal whether there is bony involvement and if so, how much and to which structures. A fine-needle aspiration biopsy would provide sufficient material for microbiological culture and antibiotic sensitivity testing; the remaining biopsy specimen would be submitted for histopathological processing and examination.

The radiograph (**169b**) revealed moderate focal osteolysis and reactive new bone formation (white arrows).

Microscopic examination of stained sections (**169c**) disclosed typical pyogranulomatous inflammation. Note the necrotic center, a band of mixed heterophilic granulocytes and histiocytic macrophages and lipid-laden cells at the outer edge of the lesion.

iii. The skink was anesthetized and the operative site prepared for aseptic surgery. The granuloma was excised from the mandible, the base was curetted, removing as much of the mandibular reactive bone as possible, and the surgical wound was left un-sutured to permit daily flushing. A broad-spectrum antibiotic was administered daily for three weeks along with parenteral physiological fluids for eight days, at which time the lizard was eating and drinking voluntarily. At 8 months, there was no recurrence and the lizard was well.

iv. The prognosis is favorable. There is always a possibility for recurrence due to the reactivation of one or more remnants of infective material; however, in this instance, the patient remained healthy.

170 Water-moistened disposable latex or nitrile plastic gloves should always be worn when handling amphibians. These moist gloves protect the amphibian's delicate skin from dermal abrasions arising from contact with the handler's fingers. The skin of amphibians is naturally protected by the lubricating mucus, which besides providing abrasion resistance, also contains immunoglobulins against many pathogens. Of course, when handling amphibians known to possess toxic secretions, protective wet gloves provide equal safety to patient and care-giver. Lastly, some/many large frogs have sharp teeth and can bite.

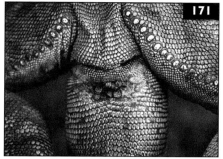

171 What is your interpretation/diagnosis of the lizard shown in Figure 171?

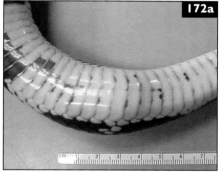

172 Figure 172a shows a California king snake (*Lampropeltis getulus californiae*) with a swelling in its caudal coelom. This swelling had been gradually increasing in size for 2 months before its owner presented the snake for examination.
i. What are some provisional diagnoses?
ii. How would you confirm your diagnosis?
iii. Depending upon your answer, how would you treat this snake?
iv. What is the prognosis?

171 Tick infestation caudal to the cloacal vent.

172 i. The swelling could be an inflammatory lesion such as an abscess or pyogranuloma, neoplasm or one or more parasitic bladder-like cysts, possibly from a cestode. When involving a king snake, milk snake (*Lampropeltis* sp.) or rattlesnake (*Crotalus* sp.), the cestode is often *Mesocestoides* sp. The swelling could also be a cystic collection of fluid from an internal organ such as the liver, kidney, ovary, a posterior abdominal aortic aneurysm, etc.

ii. Diagnostic procedures that would be helpful in determining the nature of the swelling include any or all of the following:
- Radiography.
- Ultrasonography.
- Doppler blood-flow ultrasonography.
- Fine-needle aspirate biopsy, followed by cytology and histopathology. If bladder-like hydatid cysts are suspected, an aspirate fine-needle biopsy is **contra-indicated** because of the risk of (a) anaphylaxis from cyst content spillage, or (b) release of 'daughter' cysts into the coelomic cavity.
- If deemed necessary, celioscopy or an open biopsy via a celiotomy incision.

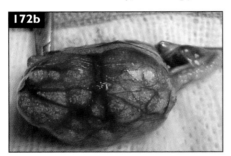

Fine-needle biopsy and histopathology revealed the mass to be a renal tubular adenoma. The snake was anesthetized, prepared for aseptic surgery, and the affected kidney was removed via a flank celiotomy (**172b**, **172c**). The characteristic histopathological features of this tumor are shown in Figure **172d**.

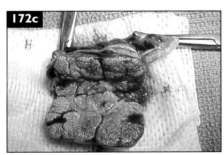

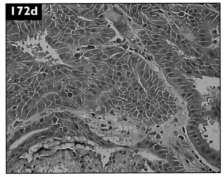

172d Renal tubular adenoma.

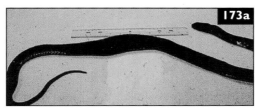

173 Figure 173a shows a spitting cobra (*Naja nigricollis*) with a marked swelling in its posterior mid-body. The snake had been on exhibit for many years and the swelling had been noted to be slowly growing for several months. (This case was selected because of one unique feature which will be discussed at the end of the answer.)

i. What are some provisional diagnoses?

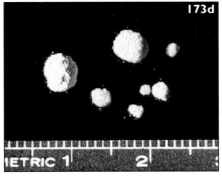

173 (*continued*) During the complete necropsy of the cobra, seven objects were identified within a cystic structure immediately caudal to the testicular tumor (173d). Analysis of these objects revealed that they were composed almost entirely of potassium ammonium urate.

ii. Accepting the fact that snakes lack a urinary bladder, how do you explain the presence of seven urinary calculi in this snake?

Answer: 173

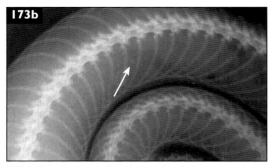

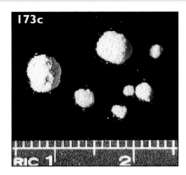

173b Dorso-ventral radiograph of the cobra. Arrow points to the larger of several radio-opaque densities within the coelomic cavity in the posterior two-thirds of the body length.

173 i. Provisional diagnoses for the swelling include the following:
• A neoplasm of an internal organ.
• An inflammatory lesion such as an abscess or pyogranuloma.
• A cystic structure in a visceral organ such as kidney, liver or gonad.
• One or more cystic hydatid-like bladder cysts arising from visceral involvement of a cestode parasite.
• A vascular lesion such as an aneurysm; unlikely but possible.

A whole-body dorso-ventral radiograph was obtained of this highly venomous snake (**173b**).

At the request of the owner, the snake was euthanized and a necropsy was performed (**173c**).

The confirmed diagnosis was Sertoli cell tumor of one testis.

173 ii. The testicular Sertoli cell tumor had grown to a size that it had exerted external pressure on the ureter to the point where urinary excretory flow was at least partially impeded; some flow must have been occurring because the kidney was not hydronephrotic. After a time, urates accumulated and eventually formed in the dilated ureter, creating a pseudobladder that permitted the formation of the discrete urinary calculi shown in Figure **173d**. It is likely that the Sertoli tumor was located in the contralateral testis. Instances of urinary calculosis in snakes are rare, but have been reported.

174 What is your diagnosis of the chelonian shown in Figure 174?

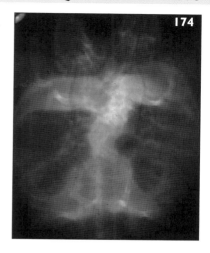

175 The red-eared slider turtles (*Trachemys scripta elegans*) shown in Figure 175 had lived almost all of their lives in the Midlands region of the UK. The turtle on the right is obviously substantially different from the one on the left.

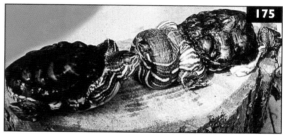

Specifically, the soft tissues comprising the skin of the neck and forequarters are enormously swollen; the limbs are not flexed as are those of the other turtle; and the animal is sluggish, to the point where it was clinically depressed.
i. With the information provided above, what is your diagnosis?

176 Figure 176 is a radiograph of a mature California desert tortoise (*Xerobates [Gopherus] agassizi*).
i. How would you treat or manage this patient for its acquired medical condition?

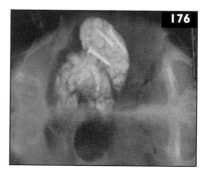

174 Unilateral pneumonia in a bicephalic (two-headed) turtle.

175 i. The differential diagnosis includes hypothyroidism. The major clues were:
- The swelling of soft tissues, which were manifestations of myxedema.
- The sluggishness, together with the marked myxedema.
- The Midlands region of the UK is very similar to the Great Lakes area of North America, in that both were considered to be geographic 'goiter belts' inasmuch as historically many humans and animals experienced hypothyroidism. For humans living in these regions, iodine is supplemented in the diet with iodized table salt.

176 i. This tortoise has ingested gravel and three metallic screws that are now admixed with other ingested radio-opaque material in its caudal intestinal tract. Although it might be possible to use stool softeners and volumes of warm water instilled into the colon by enema, there is ample reason not to do so because the sharp ends of the screws pose a threat to the delicate tissues of the colon and rectum as they pass through these organs. In this instance, a safer and more effective means for evacuating the screws and other foreign material within the colon would be via a celiotomy incision made though the plastron, thus exposing the feces and foreign objects within the colon directly so that one or more colotomy incisions can be made under direct visual observation.

NOTE: it is the author's practice that when performing a colotomy for the removal of ingested metallic foreign bodies, the feces and other material removed are placed on waxed paper and then radiographed to ensure that each and every object that was seen on the preoperative radiograph is identified and accounted for, prior to closing of the incision.

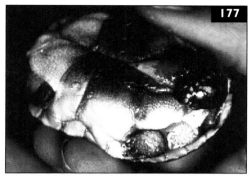

177 What is the diagnosis and terminology for the appearance of this juvenile California desert tortoise (*Xerobates [Gopherus] agassizi*) (**177**)?

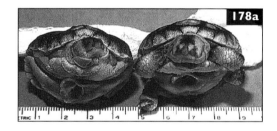

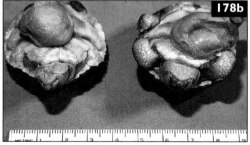

178 Figures **178a, 178b** show two recent hatchling California desert tortoise (*Xerobates [Gopherus] agassizi*) siblings. One has multiple developmental anomalies. Its sibling is normal except for one similar defect. In Figure **178b**, the yolk sacs are still attached.
i. What is your interpretation/diagnosis of these two hatchling tortoises?
ii. What is the etiology of such developmental defects?

177 Attached to the caudal end of the fresh umbilicus is a diminished parasitic twin that failed to develop. Once the dead twin is surgically removed, the larger tortoise should grow normally. This developmental anomaly is rare.

178 i. The tortoise on the left has quadrilateral fore-limb agenesis, bilateral anophthalmia and bilateral harelip defects. Its sibling clutch-mate on the right possesses all of its limbs but, like its sibling, has bilateral harelip defects.
ii. These and other developmental anomalies are commonly observed in chelonian offspring hatching from artificially incubated eggs warmed at elevated temperatures. Under natural conditions, a gravid female tortoise excavates a nest in soil and deposits her eggs one at a time in a group that falls by gravity into the nest chamber. She then back-fills the soil and often deposits urine onto the egg clutch. This urine deposition provides moisture and is also thought to deter predation by altering the scent of the egg clutch within the nest chamber. The eggs are naturally incubated, with some eggs at the periphery of the clutch being warmer or cooler, depending on the nature of the nesting medium and environmental conditions, than those in the center. This is particularly important in the biology of many chelonians – and all crocodilians – because their gender is determined epigenetically, rather than by heritable genetic heterogametic means. Eggs will produce males or females, depending upon the temperature at which they are incubated. It is well documented that excessively warm incubation temperatures can cause multiple birth defects in reptiles. This case demonstrates the range of developmental anomalies that can be induced.

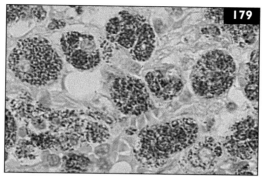

179 Fite's modified acid-fast stained mycobacteria engulfed within histiocytic macrophages.

179 Figure **179** is a photomicrograph of a histological section from a tortoise in which *Mycobacterium* sp. was isolated. In this photomicrograph numerous large phagocytic histiocytic macrophages can be seen with a myriad number of engulfed acid-fast mycobacteria within their cytoplasms.
i. How do these bacteria escape destruction and, thus, remain viable – and infective – within these leukocytes?

180 Figure **180** is a whole-body radiograph of a leopard gecko (*Eublepharis macularius*).
i. What is your diagnosis?
ii. How would you treat this patient for the problem(s) that you diagnosed?
iii. How would you prevent this from recurring or happening to other leopard geckos?

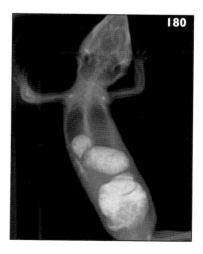

179 i. These bacteria escape phagocytic intracytoplasmic destruction because their cell walls contain a waxy substance that effectively protects them from lysis by the macrophages' lysosomal enzymes.

180 i. This lizard's gastrointestinal tract is filled with fine granular, radio-opaque material, most likely sand that it has ingested from its cage litter. Also, its skeleton exhibits osteopenia with one folding-type fracture of the left radius and bilateral ulnar curvatures.

ii. The sand can be removed by administering lactulose orally to this lizard via both a lubricated small diameter soft rubber catheter, and also its copradeum via a similar lubricated catheter introduced very gently into the cloacal vent and advanced gently and slowly until resistance is encountered. The lactulose is instilled slowly and the belly is very gently massaged. This may have to be done several times to evacuate the sand entirely. The gecko's diet should be changed to one that contains adequate calcium without excessive phosphorus, with a Ca:P content of at least 2:1. These popular lizard pets will usually avidly accept fruit nectar to which a calcium–vitamin D-3 supplement can be added.

iii. The cage litter should be changed to one that will not induce impactions if it is swallowed. Feeding dishes or cups should not be placed directly upon any particulate cage litter material.

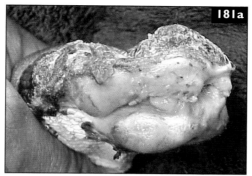

181 i. What is your interpretation/diagnosis of the condition of the South American boa constrictor (*Boa c. constrictor*) shown in Figure **181a**?

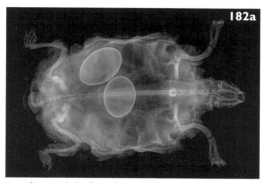

182 Figure **182a** is of an adult female African pancake tortoise (*Malacochersus tornei*), that had been straining as if to defecate for several days. The history provided by its owner confirmed that this tortoise had successfully deposited two eggs the previous year.
i. How would you treat or manage this patient?

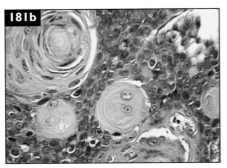

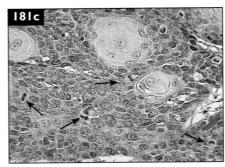

181 i. Squamous cell carcinoma (see Figures **181b, 181c**). Note the numerous mitotic figures in Figure **181c** (arrows).

182 i. The radiograph revealed that the two ova had well mineralized shells and their cross-sectional diameters were not so large as to be incapable of passing through the pelvic canal. The tortoise was administered an injection of calcium gluconate solution intracoelomically, which was followed in 40 minutes by an intramuscular injection of oxytocin dosed at 2 U/100 g body weight. Figures **182b** and **182c** were recorded 65 and 68 minutes later, respectively.

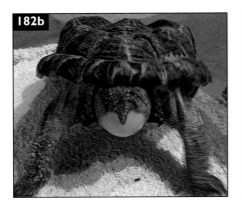

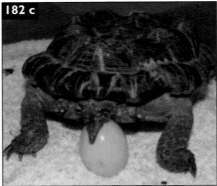

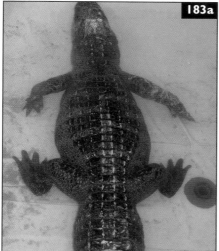

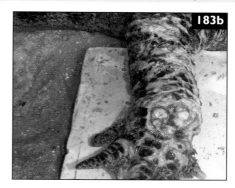

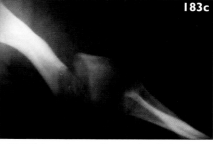

183 Figure **183a** illustrates an American alligator (*Alligator mississippiensis*) that had been in a fight with one of its tank-mates and sustained very severe bite-wound trauma to its right fore-

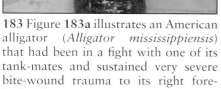

limb. The gross appearance of the wounds (**183b**) and a radiograph of the bone damage (**183c**) are shown.

i. How would you treat/manage this patient?

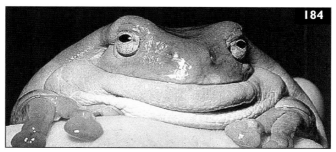

184 i. Identify this commonly kept 'pet' amphibian (**184**).

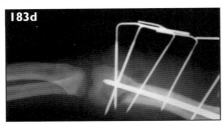

183d Postoperative radiograph obtained approximately 2 weeks after surgical repair of the right humeral fractures. There is satisfactory alignment and stabilization of the fractured humeral fragments.

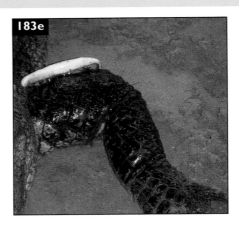

183 i. Treatment must first be directed toward cleansing the multiple bite wounds and keeping the alligator as quiescent as possible to avoid further trauma to its severely damaged limb. It should be kept 'dry-docked' in order to reduce the likelihood of further contamination, maceration and infection. Once the soft-tissue wounds are treated adequately, attention can be given to stabilizing the skeletal damage and preventing further injury. Fortunately, American alligators are relatively tractable – at least when compared with crocodiles – thus, it is somewhat safer for the personnel responsible for their care.

The veterinarian in this case performed open reduction, employing both an intramedullary pin in the humerus and smaller pins to help stabilize and further bring the distal humeral fragment into anatomical apposition. The smaller pins were bent to a right angle and then secured in place with a plastic resin splint that encapsulated each of the pins, therefore ensuring that movement of the pins and the fragments that they held would not shift, thus enhancing the chance for primary uinion of the fragments of bone that they held in place (**183d**). The alligator was provided antibiotic coverage administered via intramuscular injections and topical application of a broad-spectrum bacterio*cidal* antibiotic ointment.

This was a particularly difficult case that was managed brilliantly and had a good outcome (**183e**).

184 i. White's tree frog, *Litoria caerulea*.

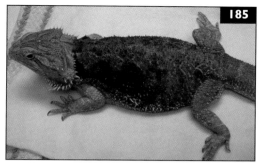

185 i. What is your diagnosis of this bearded dragon lizard's (*Pogona vitticeps*) medical condition (**185**)?
ii. How would you confirm your diagnosis?
iii. How would you treat this lizard?

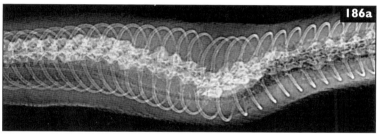

186 i. What is your diagnosis of the medical condition affecting this snake (**186a**)?
ii. What is the prognosis for this snake?

185 i. The bearded dragon lizard appears to have a pigmented dermatopathy covering an expanse of its left dorsum. Additional lesions were located on the belly. These lesions could be of bacterial or mycotic (fungal) origin.

ii. Appropriate specimens of the active lesion should be submitted for cytology, bacterial culture and sensitivity testing, as well as fungal culture and characterization. A dermatophyte test vial, containing fungal culture with a test dye to signal a positive test reaction, is a quick and convenient means for determining in-house whether a fungal pathogen is present and is relatively inexpensive. However, characterization and taxonomic assignment usually requires the expertise of someone trained in medical mycology.

iii. Depending upon results of microbiological culture, an appropriate topical and/or parenteral antibiotic or antifungal medication should be administered. In this instance, the fungal culture grew out *Microsporum caninum* and no other pathogens. The treatment was a course of topical ketoconazole. Any of several alternative antimycotic agents could have been selected.

186 i. At first glance, this snake exhibits multifocal exostoses involving its vertebral column. These osseous excrescences do not appear to involve the ribs. These features are characteristic of osteitis deformans (Paget's disease of bone). However, in order to evaluate more fully this snake's spinal osteopathology, a radiograph with a orthogonal view should be obtained (**186b**). The displaced vertebral fracture can be readily appreciated.

ii. The prognosis is grave because of the displacement and probable spinal cord disruption.

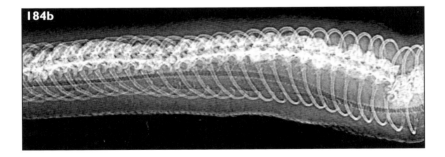

184b

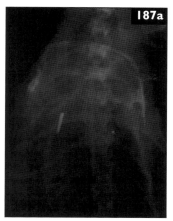

187 What is your interpretation/diagnosis of this dorso-ventral radiograph if a wild-caught Cuban rock iguana, *Cyclura nubila* (187a)?

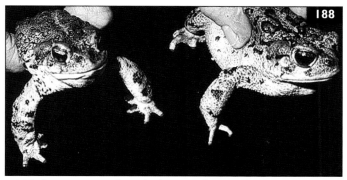

188 Figure 188 shows a pair of spade-foot toads, *Scaphiopus* sp. Which is the male of this pair?

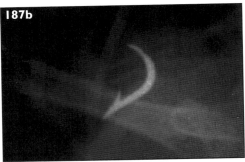

187 There is a radio-opaque foreign object in the left anterior thoracic portion of the coelom.

A lateral projection radiograph is shown (**187b**). Note the fish hook as viewed from the side. This case exemplifies the value of taking orthogonal views.

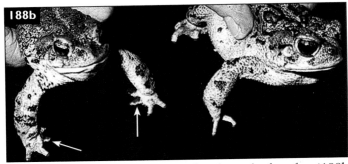

188 The male is on the left. Note the nuptial pads on the fore-feet (**188b**, arrows).

These roughened dermal callosities are employed to hold the female during amplexus (copulatory embrace).

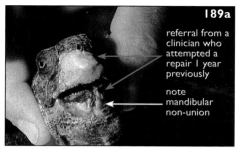

189a

referral from a
clinician who
attempted a
repair 1 year
previously

note
mandibular
non-union

189 Figure **189a** shows an adult desert tortoise (*Xerobates [Gopherus] agassizi*) that was referred for evaluation approximately 1 year after it was treated for maxillary and mandibular symphyseal fractures. Both fractures had failed to unite after an attempt to stabilize the fracture sites with an orthopedic wire in the rostrum, but no additional support in the mandible. Cold-setting dental acrylic cement was used to cover both fracture sites. The fractures probably failed to unite because of lack of fixation and the resulting motion at both fractures sites.
i. How would you treat/manage this patient to affect a permanent bony union?

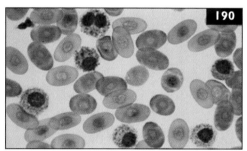

190

190 What is your diagnosis of the stained blood film from a green iguana (*Iguana iguana*) shown in Figure **190**?

189 i. The tortoise was sedated and the operative sites were prepared for aseptic surgery after the dental acrylic splints were removed with a rotating dental burr. Both the maxillary and mandibular symphyseal fractures were found to be loose with no evidence of fracture callus formation. After the edges of both fractures were freshened, paired Kirschner orthopedic pins were inserted in the mandibular fracture site (arrows) and the wire that was previously placed in the maxillary rostrum was tightened. Both procedures stabilized the two fractures. After the ends of these pins were cut with approximately 1.5–2.0 mm extending beyond the surfaces of the right and left sides, they were covered with freshly prepared cold-setting dental acrylic cement (**189b–f**).

An abrasive emery board was used to create a sharp cutting edge on the outer surface of the mandibular repair so that the tortoise could bite pieces of vegetation free before attempting to swallow them (**189g**).

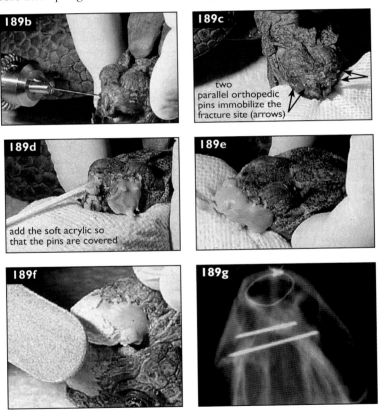

190 Azurophilic leukemia. Note the marked anisocytosis, aniso-nucleocytosis and binucleated azuroblast.

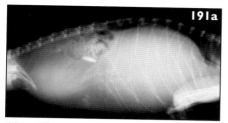
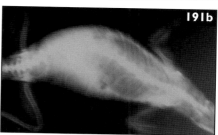

191 Figures 191a, 191b illustrate
an 8-year-old female green iguana (*Iguana iguana*) that had developed a slowly
growing and firm swelling of its abdomen. She had exhibited polydipsia for 1
month. Her history revealed that she had deposited eggs for several years in the
past. Upon examination significant abdominal distention, muscle wasting and
dehydration were noted.

i. How would you investigate the etiology of this swelling in order to formulate a
provisional diagnosis?

The following are pertinent laboratory findings from blood:

WBC	13,500/mm^3 (13.5 × 10^9/l)
Heterophils	56%
Lymphocytes	15%
Azurophils	14%
Monocytes	13%
Basophils	2%
PCV	27%
Polychromasia	+1
Total protein	3.4 g/dl (34 g/l)
Globulin	2.3 g/dl (23 g/l)
Albumin	1.1 g/dl (11 g/l)
Glucose	126 mg/dl (7 mmol/l)
SGOT (AST)	31 IU (norm = 10–50)
CPK	1,203 IU (norm = 50–400)
Calcium	8.7 mg/dl (2.2 mmol/l) (norm = 8.0–13.0 [2.0–3.3])
Phosphorus	9.8 mg/dl (3.2 mmol/l) (norm= 5.0–8.0 [1.6–2.6])
Potassium	5.0 mEq/dl (50 mmol/l) (norm = 1.5–5.5 [15–55])
Uric acid	12.7 mg/dl (0.76 mmol/l) (norm = 2.0–7.0 [0.12–0.42])

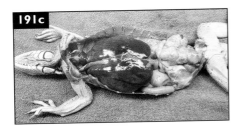

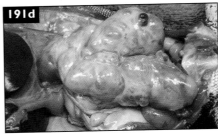

191d Ovarian mass.

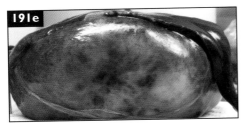

191e Mass within liver.

191 i. The iguana was examined thoroughly and while palpating its body the extent of the swelling was more fully appreciated. Lateral and dorso-ventral radiographs were obtained, which revealed that there was a radio-opaque mass occupying much of the caudal coelomic cavity. A fine-needle aspirate could have been employed, followed by cytology, culture and antibiotic sensitivity testing and histopathology, probably could have yielded an accurate diagnosis. However, at the owner's request, the iguana was euthanized and a thorough necropsy performed. Selected images recorded during that necropsy are shown (191c–e).

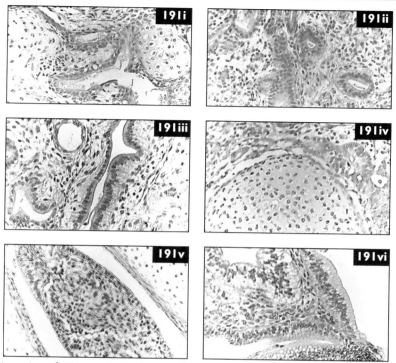

191 (*continued*) Figure **191** shows photomicrographs of the neoplastic tissues observed in the ovarian and hepatic tumors.

ii. Based solely upon the organ where this neoplasm originated, i.e. the primary site (ovary), the histopathological characteristics and its metastasis to the liver, what is your diagnosis of this neoplasm?

192 The radiograph in Figure **192a** is of the head of a boa constrictor (*Boa c. constrictor*) after it had sustained trauma while trying to subdue a large violently struggling rodent that it had grasped. The mandible was grossly distorted. An open-mouth radiographic view was made. The white arrow points to a fractured right mandibular ramus.

i. How would you treat this patient?

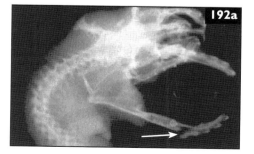

191 ii. Teratoma, malignant. These neoplasms are characterized by the presence of tissues originating from all three germ layers: entoderm, mesoderm and ectoderm. Thus tissues representing gut, pulmonary and glandular epithelial structures, smooth and skeletal muscle, myocardium, bone and cartilage, can be identified. For instance, note the ciliated pulmonary epithelium and cartilage in the first of these photomicrographs. Often, various tissue types are disorganized with respect to each other. The fact that this ovarian tumor had metastasized to the liver is confirmation of its potential for malignancy.

192i. The boa was anesthetized and the operative site was prepared for aseptic surgery. Using disposable stainless steel hypodermic needles as fixation pins, two pairs were inserted into and entirely through both sides of the mandibular fracture. Once the proper placement of the pins was assured, the pins were secured in place with cold-curing dental acrylic cement and the balance of each was cut off. Additional acrylic was added to cover the ends of each needle (**192b**). A broad-spectrum bacterio*cidal* antibiotic was administered for 10 days postoperatively as a prophylactic measure. The snake was not fed during the approximately 2 months that the mandible was healing, but fresh water was always available in its cage.

Once follow-up radiographs confirmed that the mandibular fracture had healed sufficiently, the snake was again anesthetized and the dental acrylic and repurposed cannulae/orthopedic pins were removed (**192c**). Once the pins and acrylic cement were removed, the snake was offered small killed rodents, which it accepted and ate.

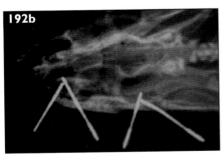

192b Immediate postoperative appearance. Note the reasonably close alignment of the mandibular fragments.

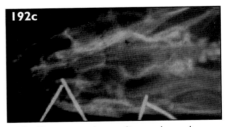

192c Postoperative radiograph made several weeks after the fracture was stabilized. Note the callus at the site of fracture, which further secured and spanned the gap in the mandible.

193 In Figure **193**, a person's fingers are holding and extending the flounce-like cervical fringe of a fringed lizard, *Clamydosaurus* sp. In so doing so, paired swellings are seen on either side of the dorsal mid-line.
i. Identify these structures.
ii. What is their function?

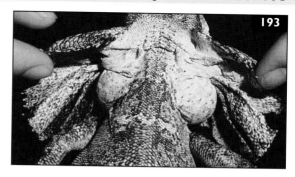

194 i. Identify the depressions along this ball (regal) python's (*Python regius*) maxillary lip margin (**194**).
ii. What is the function of these structures?

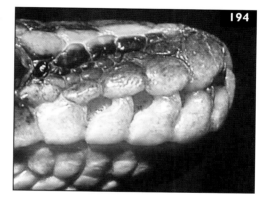

195 i. Identify the golden tan objects on the underside of this lizard's thighs and cloacal region (**195**).
ii. What is the function of these structures?

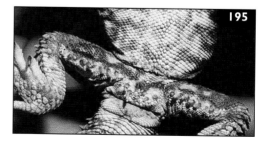

193 i. The paired softly fluctuant structures are called 'chalk sacs'.

ii. They function as a storage depot for calcium salts that can be mobilized if needed, particularly by females preparatory to producing shelled eggs. They are highly modified extensions of the endolymphatic system and are found in several lizard taxa.

194 i. They are labial pit organs.

ii. These structures are sensory organs sensitive to thermal radiation. Pit organs are capable of detecting minor changes in the thermal milieu of the snake, thus enabling detection of warm-blooded prey and, perhaps predators, at a safe distance.

195 i. The structures are femoral pores. They are integumentary modified sebaceous-like holocrine glandular organs that secrete a waxy, pheromone-rich substance that the lizards can rub onto substrates and conspecific females.

ii. They are employed by conspecific lizards as a means for communicating one another's presence, particularly when it relates to sexual activity, especially courtship and copulation.

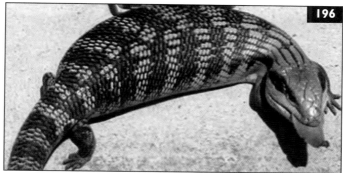

196 Identify this popular reptile 'pet' (196).

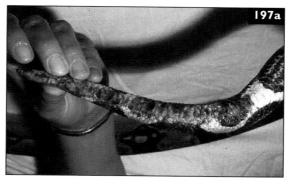

197 Bandaging snakes is often an exercise in frustration because these creatures can crawl though almost any conventional bandaging scheme. Applying adhesive tape to their skin is also not recommended except under special circumstances. Figure 197a illustrates an instance where a covering bandage would be helpful in promoting healing of a sub-acute bacterial dermatitis involving the tail of a boa constrictor.

i. How would you bandage this patient's tail?

196 Blue-tongue skink (*Tiliqua* sp.).

197 i. Placing a non-lubricated condom filled with a water soluble (NOT oil-soluble) ointment has proven very effective as a medicated dressing in cases such as this one. Figures **197b–d** illustrate how this is accomplished.

The water-soluble wound antiseptic silver sulfadiazine is placed in the tip of the unrolled condom (**197b**, black arrows) and is then rolled up and over the tail tip (**197c**).

It is important to trim the short length of elastic adhesive tape to a curvilinear shape so that it will not catch on cage surfaces and become detached. Figure **197d** image was recorded 7 days after the condom was placed on the tail lesion.

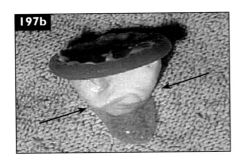

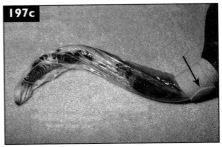

197c Cut the end of the elastic adhesive tape with a round edge. Cutting it square will cause it to catch on cage surfaces and/or unravel, thus loosening it. Unroll the condom and massage onto and over the surfaces of the affected skin.

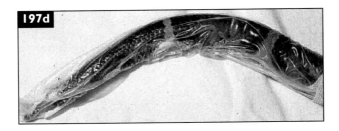

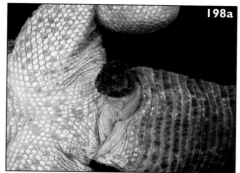

198 Figure **198a** shows the cloacal region of a male monitor lizard that suffered a prolapse of the left hemipenis 2 weeks previously. The prolapsed copulatory organ was necrotic and desiccated.

i. How would you manage this patient?

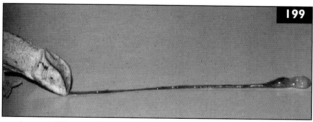

199 The chameleon (*Chamaeleo* sp.) shown in Figure **199** has developed lingual paralysis and, therefore, presents a special challenge to a veterinarian engaged in herpetological medicine and surgery. These lizards use their projectile tongue with its sticky tip for capturing insect prey before swallowing them.

i. How would you manage this patient?

ii. What is the prognosis for this animal's survival in captivity?

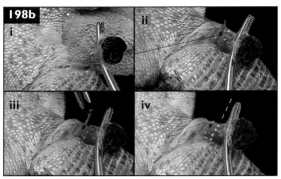

198b (i–iv) Technique for hemipenial amputation.

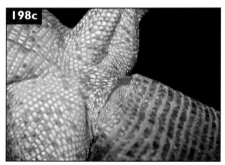

198c Immediate postoperative appearance.

198 i. The necrotic hemipenis should be amputated. Because these organs are paired, it is possible this lizard will still be able to breed. Figure **198b** illustrate the technique for hemipenial amputation.

NOTE: traction is exerted on the prolapsed hemipenis and a circumferential ligating suture is placed through and around the base of the organ; the suture is then transfixed by passing the needle entirely through the organ to ensure that the ligature cannot slip off of the stump. The tissue is then excised. Once the mild traction is released, the stump retracts back into its sulcus within the base of the tail (**198c**).

199 i. The tongue must be amputated. After general anesthesia, gentle traction is applied to the chameleon's tongue in order to gain access to as much of its caudal attachment as possible, before placing a transfixed circumferential ligature and excising it.

ii. The postoperative prognosis is favorable because these lizards can be trained to accept living invertebrate prey from the end of a forceps. Of course, they must not be released to the wild to fend for themselves because without their projectile tongue they could not capture live insect prey.

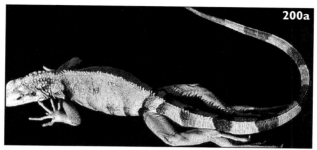

200 i. What is your impression of the adult female green iguana (*Iguana iguana*) shown in Figure **200a**?

ii. How would you investigate this case to determine the etiology of its clinical signs?

iii. How would you manage this patient?

iv. What is the prognosis?

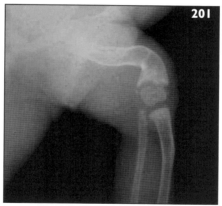

201 i. What is your diagnosis of the radiograph in Figure **201**?

ii. How would you manage this patient?

iii. What is the prognosis?

193

200 i. Note the flaccid paralysis of the hind-limbs and the normal flexion of the fore-limbs. This suggests a spinal cord lesion.

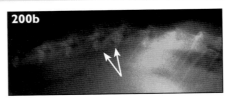

ii. The iguana had a greatly diminished toe pinch response and no pain response to needle pricks applied to its hind-limbs. A radiograph of the spine revealed two compression fractures of the iguana's lumbar vertebrae (200b, arrows).

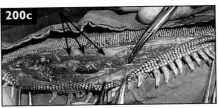

iii. Following initial stabilization, the iguana was anesthetized and a laminectomy was performed on the two crushed vertebrae, as well as the ones immediately cranial and caudal to the sites of compression fractures, 'unroofing' the dorsal spinal canal over the area of spinal cord damage (200c).

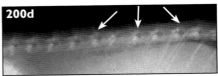

Prior to surgery and afterward, the iguana was administered intravenous mannitol solution, a corticoseroid and a bactero*cidal* antibiotic.

A postoperative radiograph showing area of laminectomy of the last thoracic and first three lumbar vertebrae (white arrows) is shown in Figure 200d.

iv. The prognosis was guarded. However, the iguana was regaining the use of its hind-limbs when it died as a result of a bile duct carcinoma. This was a cause unrelated to its vertebral spinal trauma.

NOTE: this was a highly unusual case inasmuch as the owner of the iguana was not only very fond of his pet and was also able and willing to pay the significant fees for treating it, rather than euthanizing it. This case illustrates what *can* be done when all of the various factors that are essential for success are in place.

201 i. A pseudoarthrosis (false joint) has formed at the fracture site of the deformed distal femur and tibial–fibular articulation.

ii. At this point, there would be little to gain by intervening; the pseudoarthrosis permits the animal to ambulate.

iii. The prognosis is favorable without further professional care for this chronic condition.

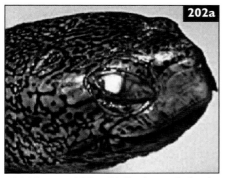 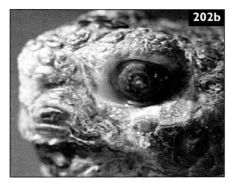

202 Figures **202a, 202b** show chelonians that, after awakening from hibernation, were found to have accumulations of tenacious proteinaceous exudate adhering to their corneas.
i. How would you remove these accumulations safely and effectively?

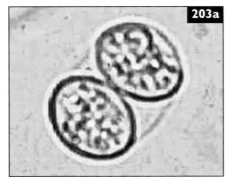

203 Identify this organism found while performing a fecal examination on a monitor lizard (*Varanus* sp.) (**203a**).

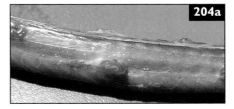

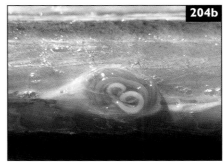

204 Figures **204a, 204b** were recorded during the necropsy of a European snake, the taxonomy of which is unknown.
i. Identify the encysted helminthes exposed when the snake's skin was removed.

202 i. These plaques of exudate can be safely and effectively removed from the corneas by applying the plant enzyme, papain, either as a diluted solution of papain powder or as a small piece of papaya fruit cut freshly and applied to the affected eye(s). This enzyme is chemically active at relatively low temperatures, whereas commercial enzymatic preparations designed for humans and other mammals are active at only substantially higher (body) temperatures.

203 *Sarcocystis* sp. Note the delicate membrane encircling the paired cysts (**203b**).

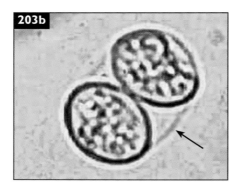

204 i. *Dracunculus* sp.

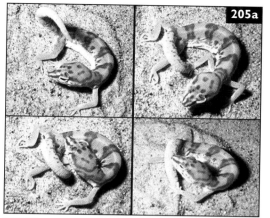
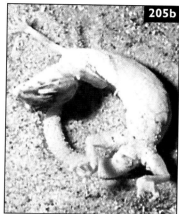

205 Figures **205a, 205b** record the behavior of a gecko, *Coleonyx* sp. These events repeated themselves every few minutes.
i. What are some plausible diagnoses?

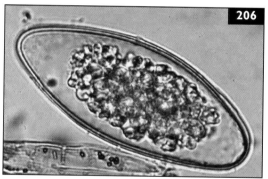

206 Identify this ovum discovered while performing a fecal examination on a reticulated python (*Python reticulatus*) (**206**).

197

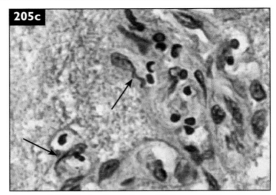

205 i. There are signs of CNS dysfunction. This could be due to an inflammatory process, a space-occupying lesion, a metabolic derangement or an intoxication by an environmental agent. Because the prognosis was poor, the owner elected to have the gecko euthanized and permitted a necropsy to be performed. A photomicrograph of a stained histological section of this lizard's brain is shown (205c). Note the trypanosome mastigotes (arrows).

206 *Ophiostrongylus* sp.

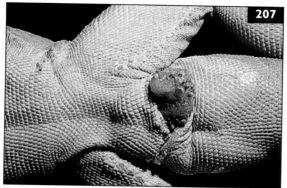

207 Figure 207 shows a young male green iguana (*Iguana iguana*).
i. What is your diagnosis?
ii. What environmental factors contributed to this condition?
iii. How would you treat this patient?
iv. What recommendations can you make to help avoid this condition?

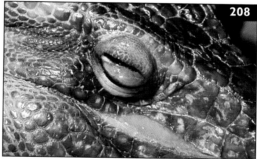

208 The red tegu lizard (*Tupinambis rufescens*) shown in Figure 208 has severe blepharitis induced by which of these vitamin deficiencies: A, thiamine; B, pantothenic acid; C, vitamin D-3; D, vitamin A?

207 i. Balanoposthitis and mechanical paraphimosis involving the left hemipene.
ii. In this instance, the coarse abrasive sand that was furnished as cage substrate has adhered to the moist delicate hemipenial tissues and has impeded the retraction of the organ.
iii. Treatment is gentle lavage to remove the particles of sand. Once cleaned and sand-free, a lubricating ointment was applied to the prolapsed hemipenis and the organ was replaced into its sulcus.
iv. Iguanas are normally arboreal lizards and thus live much of their time in trees. The sand substrate should be changed to something less likely to adhere to moist body surfaces. Parenthetically, sand substrates have also been implicated in impactions of lizards maintained in cages with this substance as a material in which they can burrow. Fine silica sand can also be ingested directly with moist food items to which it adheres as the animals swallow their food.

208 D, vitamin A.

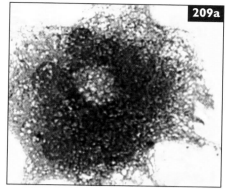

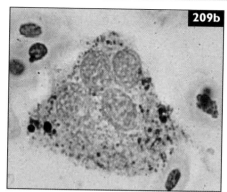

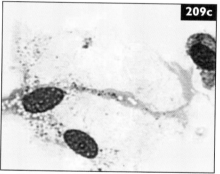

209 Figures **209a**, **209b** show multinucleated cells that were observed in a blood film from a green iguana (*Iguana iguana*). Figure **209a** was stained with Wright's stain; Figure **209b** with Megacolor.

Figure **209c** was recorded after one of these multinucleated cells was gently teased apart prior to staining with Wright's stain.

i. Identify the multinucleated cells.

ii. To what do these multinucleated cells give rise to in the peripheral blood?

iii. What is the function of these individual cells?

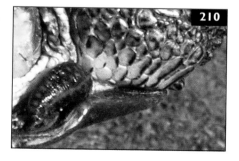

210 What is your diagnosis of this Pacific pond turtle's (*Arctemys marmorata*) condition (**210**)?

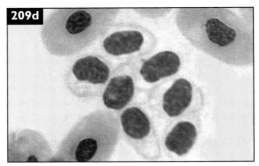

209d A raft of thrombocytes among several mature erythrocytes.

209 i. The multinucleated cells are megakaryocytes.
ii. They give rise to thrombocytes (Figure **209d**).
iii. Thrombocytes are essential for blood clotting and under certain circumstances, can perform as phagocytes of particulate matter.

210 Parasitism by a leech, *Placabdella* sp. attached to the turtle's axilla.

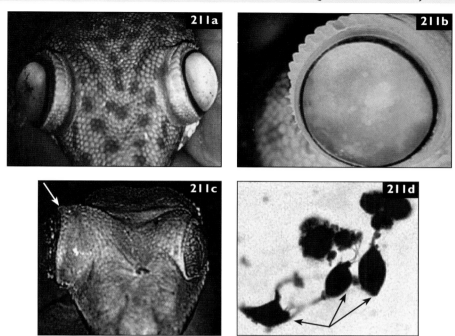

211 Figures **211a, 211b** show the eyes of a Tokay gecko (*Gekko gecko*). The eyes are swollen and opaque.

Figure **211c** is an image of another Tokay gecko from the same collection. This gecko displayed unilateral swelling (arrow)

The lizard's eye was prepared for an aseptic needle aspiration and a sample of exudate was withdrawn for cytology and microbiological culture and sensitivity testing. A stained preparation was made from that exudate, shown in Figure **211d**.
i. What is your diagnosis of the objects (indicated by black arrows)?

212 The arrow in Figure **212a** is pointing to an object lying within the conjunctival sac and across the lower surface of the cornea of an African Nile monitor lizard (*Varanus niloticus*).
i. What is your interpretation/diagnosis?

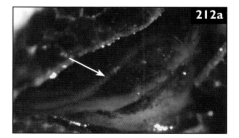

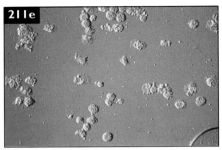 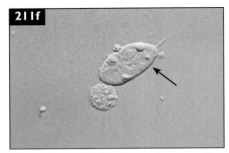

211 i. Trichomonads; the diagnosis is ocular trichomoniasis. Once the organism was identified, the balance of the aspirate was inoculated onto a special growth medium. A few days later, colonies had formed on the growth medium (**211e, 211f**).

212 i. The 'object' is an adult rhabdidiform helminth (**212b**).

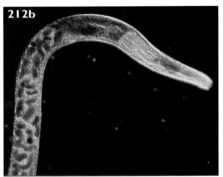

212b Nematode recovered from lizard's conjunctiva.

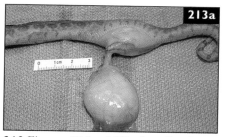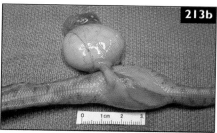

213 Figures **213a, 213b** describe the surgery on a neonate python.
i. What is your diagnosis?
ii. How would you manage this patient?
iii. What is the prognosis?

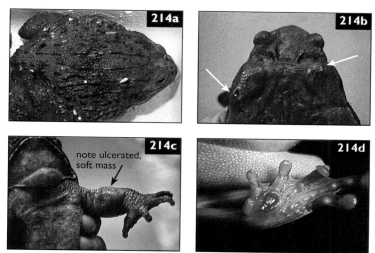

214 Four diffferent amphibians with ulcerative dermal lesions are shown in Figures **214a–d**. These dermatopathies are commonly encountered in captive amphibians.
i. The pathogenic microorganisms most frequenlty cultured from these ulcerative lesions are which of the following:
A, *Streptococcus* sp.;
B, *Enterobacter* sp.;
C, *Aeromonas* sp.;
D, *Lactobacilus* sp.?

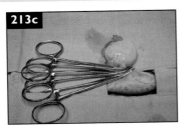

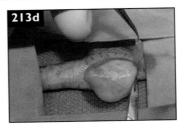

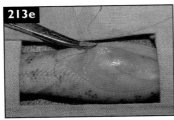

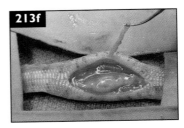

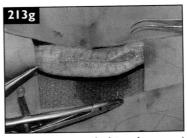

213 i. The python hatchling has a omphalocoele containing the yolk sac; there was also segmental agenesis of the integument surrounding the periumbilical body wall defect.

ii. Figures **213c–g** illustrates the surgical repair of this developmental anomaly.

The yolk sac remnant and omphalocoel were cross-clamped and double-ligated. Then the area of dermal agenesis was excised to provide a site for suturing the body wall to provide normal support for the viscera contained within the coelom. The two freshened edges of the body wall were then united by careful suturing. The site of the belly wall repair lacked a section of belly scutes, but, despite this, the snake was able to crawl normally after the surgery.

iii. The prognosis is favorable.

214 i. C, *Aeromonas* sp.

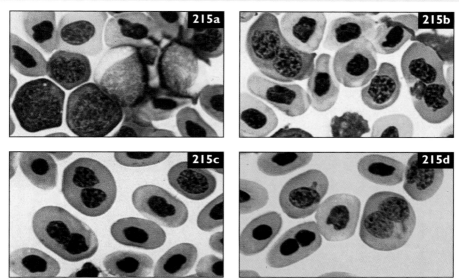

215 Figures 215a–d shows stained blood films made from a mature green iguana (*Iguana iguana*) that had a history of gradual onset of lethargy, weight loss and exhaustion after even mild exertion.
i. After examining the photomicrographs, what is your provisional diagnosis?

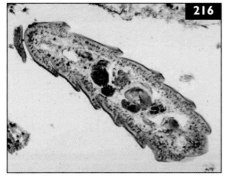

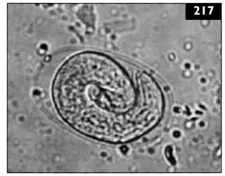

216 i. Identify the helminth revealed while examining this stained histologic section (216).
ii. Does this parasite utilize a direct or indirect life cycle?

217 Identify the embryonated helminth ovum in Figure 217.

215 i. Erythroleukemia. Note the marked anisocytosis, large basophilic erythroblasts with prominent nuclei, increased mitotic activity, numerous binucleated erythrocytes and polychromatophilia. These are all evidence of dedifferentiation of previously committed mature cells.

216 i. A cestode (tapeworm).
ii. An indirect life cycle, involving at least one, and sometimes multiple intermediate hosts.

217 The correct identification of such embryonated ova depends upon the animal from whose feces are being examined. The correct identification could be any of the following:
If the host was a snake:
• *Rhabdias* sp.
• *Acanthorhabdias* sp.
• *Strongyloides* sp.
• *Kalicephalus* sp.

If the host was a lizard:
• *Strongyloides* sp.
• *Shorttia* sp.
• *Entomelas* sp.

If the host was a chelonian:
• *Chapinella* sp.

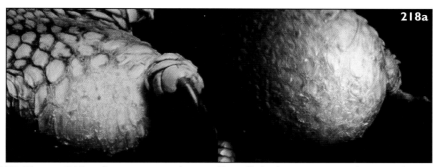

218 Figure **218a** shows a grossly swollen digit from a green iguana (*Iguana iguana*). Preliminary investigation revealed that the toe was massively abscessed.
i. How would you manage this patient?

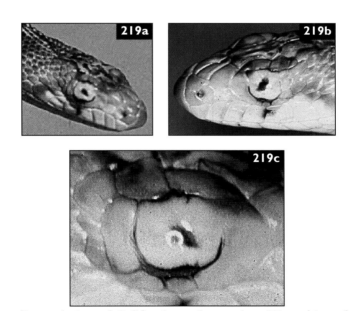

219 A small population of California gopher snakes (*Pituophis melanoleucus catenifer*) has developed, very probably through the action of a point mutation, a sub-lethal genetic developmental anomaly that affects their eyes. Examples of this anomaly are shown (**219a–c**).
i. What is your interpretation of this lesion?

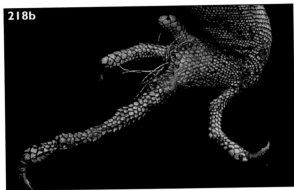

218 i. The digit was not only superficially infected, but the distal phalanx was also involved. Thus a decision to amputate the entire digit was made in such a fashion that the result would be cosmetically acceptable. Figure **218b** shows the postoperative result. Once the sutures were removed, the limb was fully functional and few people would notice that the digit was missing.

219 i. Unlike dermatization of the tertiary spectacles that was shown in an earlier case (27) in a python, this was dermatization of the *cornea*; the spectacles of these snakes are normal and shed without problems. These snakes survive in their native habitat.

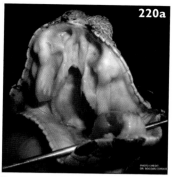
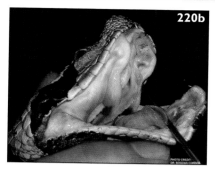

220 Figures **220a, 220b** show a mature Gaboon viper (*Bitis gabonicus*) as it was presented for evaluation by its owner. The snake was a long-term captive in a collection. The only important item of its history given by the owner was that the snake had recently tried to kill but had failed to envenomate mice that were introduced into its cage.

i. What is your diagnosis?
ii. How would you manage this patient?
iii. What is your prognosis?
iv. If this was a recently captured wild snake, what else should be considered?

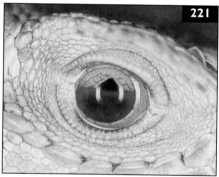

221 What is your interpretation/diagnosis of the iguana shown in Figure **221**?

220 i. The snake has ulcerative stomatitis and appears to have lost its fangs, or at least one may be incarcerated in inflamed and significantly swollen fang sheath tissue.

ii. The snake should be administered a bacterio*cidal* broad-spectrum antibiotic that can be injected. Even though this snake may not have functioning fangs when these images were recorded, *reserve* fangs can drop into place in a short time and, thus render this animal quite dangerous to handle. The snake can be fed pre-killed mice in lieu of living ones.

iii. The prognosis is favorable.

iv. Great care should be exercised when handling this snake, regardless of whether it has its fangs in place or not, or whether it was recently caught or a long-term captive. Reserve fangs can drop down in place within 1–2 days of their predecessors having been lost.

221 Hyphema; hemorrhage into the anterior chamber of the eye.

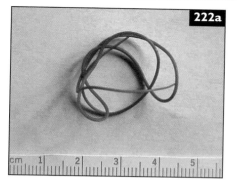

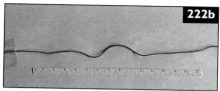

222 i. Identify the elongated organism shown in Figures **222a, 222b**. One shows it coiled, the other stretched out to its full length.

ii. Is this organism parasitic in amphibians and reptiles?

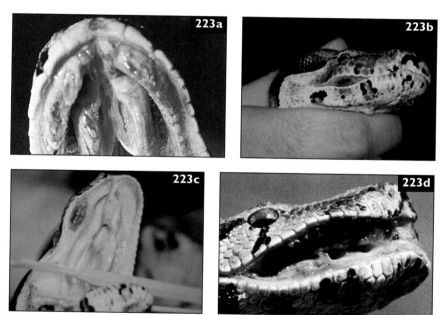

223 Figures **223a–d** show different snakes with the same infectious disease at different stages of its progression.

i. What is the condition?

ii. How would you treat it?

iii. What is the prognosis for recovery?

222 i. The organism is *Gordia* sp., also known as 'horsehair' worms (Nematomorpha) (**222c**).
ii. These organisms are not parasites of either amphibians or reptiles. Rather, they are parasites of some insects, especially grasshoppers, locusts, crickets and katydids.

223 i. Ulcerative stomatitis (commonly referred to as 'mouth rot' in lay literature).
ii. After establishing the etiologic agent and determining its antibiotic susceptibility, gentle but thorough debridement, lavaging with a non-cytotoxic wound flushing agent such as 0.75% chlorhexidine diacetate (or gluconate), parenteral broad-spectrum bacteriocidal antibiotic(s) and administration of appropriate physiologic fluid therapy to maintain renal perfusion. In addition, providing additional cage warmth is often beneficial to promote, maintain and enhance celluilar and humoral immunity.
iii. When treated aggressively, the prognosis is often favorable.

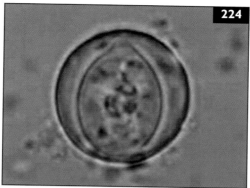

224 Identify the organism that was revealed while peforming a microscopic examination of feces from a European viper, *Vipera berus* (**224**).

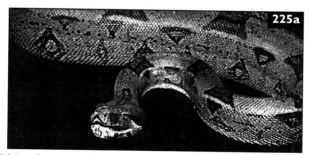

225 Figure **225a** shows an immature South American boa constrictor (*Boa c. constrictor*).
i. What is your impression and/or interpretation of this snake's physical problem?

224 *Caryospora* sp.

225 i. The boa is exhibiting respiratory distress. Note the open-mouth breathing and the evidence of inspiratory effort (Figure **225b**, white arrows).

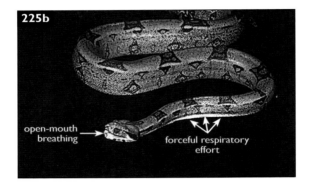

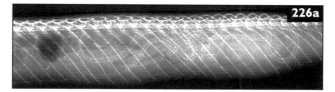

226 What is your interpretation of the following radiographs of a rattlesnake (226a, 226b)?

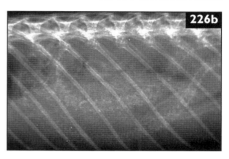

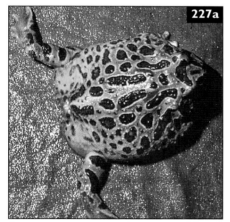

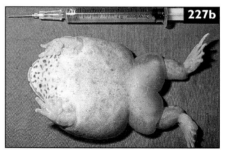

227 The Argentine horned frog (*Ceratophrys ornate*) shown in Figures 227a, 227b was referred for evaluation of its massive body swelling. The history obtained from the owner was that the frog was approximately 2 years old and its diet was small goldfish that were kept in an aquarium as feeders; these fish were fed a commercial fish food that contained a balanced vitamin–mineral formula designed for freshwater aquarium fish.

Upon initial examination the frog was found to be distended with both intracoelomic ascitic fluid, as well as severe subcutaneous edema accumulations. A fluid sample of 6 ml was withdrawn aseptically and was shown to have a specific gravity of 1.011 by refractometer.

i. Based upon this information, what organ systems do you suspect as being involved in this frog's anasarca and ascites?

226 The rattlesnake is gravid. Note the multiple skeletons within the coelomic cavity. Rattlesnakes, like most pit vipers, are ovoviviparous (live-bearing).

227 i. Any and/or all of the following organ systems could be responsible for the alarming accumulations of both ascitic as well as subcutaneous and intracoelomic fluid:
- Heart.
- Kidneys.
- Liver.
- Alimentary system (via nutritional hypoproteinemia or a protein-wasting enteropathy).
- Lymphatic drainage obstruction from either protozoan or metazoan parasitism.

Figure **227c** illustrates significant findings revealed during the necropsy and histopathological examination of stained tissue sections.

Note that the heart is spherical and has a distinctly mottled appearance. Figure **227d** is a photomicrograph of a section of renal tissue, with multiple foci of dystrophic soft-tissue mineralization indicated by arrows.

Figure **227e** is a photomicrograph of a section of myocardium from the frog, which also exhibits significant soft-tissue mineralization and intermyocardial edema.

The liver was also severly mineralized, as were some of the airways in its lungs. Thus, the explanation for this frog's various fluid accumulations can be attributed to the multifocal nature of its soft-tissue mineral deposits. Investigating this case further, the underlying etiology of this animal's soft-tissue mineralizations was traced to the fish food that was fed to the feeder fish that this frog ingested several times

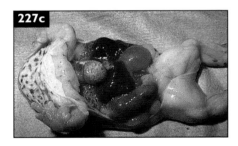

a week. The fish food's vitamin D-3 and calcium levels were substantially above those appropriate for amphibians and this induced hypervitaminosis-D-3 and hypercalcemia-related soft-tissue dystrophic mineralization.

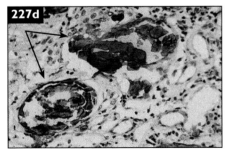

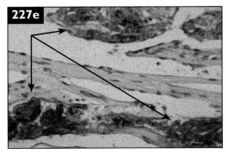

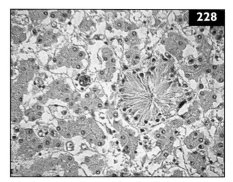

228 While examining the hepatic tissues obtained during the necropsy of an African spurred tortoise (*Geochelone sulcata*) you find the image field shown (228).
i. What is your interpretation of the 'star-burst' lesion?

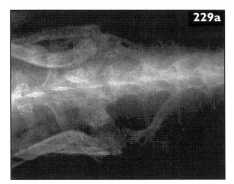

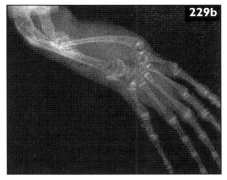

229 Figures **229a–c** illustrate the appendicular and posterior axial skeleton of an Asian water dragon (*Physignathus concincinus*) that was presented for examination and evaluation for severe lameness and reluctance to walk or swim.
i. What is your interpretation/diagnosis of this lizard's medical problem?
ii. What is the likely etiology for this condition?
iii. How would you treat this patient?
iv. What is the prognosis? Why?

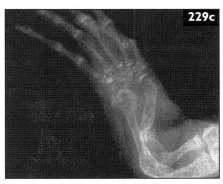

Answers: 228, 229

228 i. The 'star-burst' shaped lesion is a gouty tophus and is consistent with hyperuricemia-induced visceral gout.

229 i. Some form of metabolic osteopathy with multiple foci of osteopenia/osteoporosis, multiple folding fractures of the major long bones of the appendicular skeleton, particularly both radii, ulnae, proximal femurs and femoral capiti. Partial to complete luxations of both ulnae and radial-carpal articulations, severe osteopenia of the pelvic architecture, especially involving the pubic and and ilial sections.

ii. The etiology could be any of the following possibilities:
- Primary hyperparathyroidism, induced by a functioning parathyroid adenoma.
- Secondary nutritional hyperparathyroidism, induced by any of the following:
  o A diet deficient in available calcium content or overly rich in phosphorus, the ideal ratio being at least 2:1 Ca:P.
  o Inadequate exposure to the appropriate wavelength of UV illumination, either natural sunlight or articifical source(s) that are sufficient to permit the endosynthesis of vitamin D-3.
  o Inadequate preformed vitamin D-3 in the diet.

Renal insufficiency that permits the excretion of calcium ions in the urine and/or the retention of phosphorus ion products.

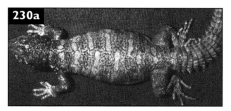

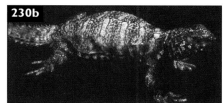

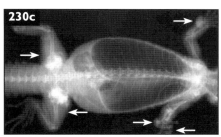

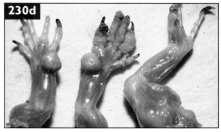

230 A long-term captive male ornate uromastyx lizard (*Uromastyx ornata*) was presented by its owner with a complaint that the lizard had gradually been reluctant to move about in its cage. The owner also stated that he had noticed that his pet had also developed multiple swellings that involved several joints. Figures 230a–c show this lizard in the stance that it had adopted; he would only move when prodded. Note the multiple swellings on the appendages. The most florid lesions were those that involved the coxo-femoral articulations and radio-carpal joints (230c, white arrows). Other than these abnormalities, there were no additional radiologically significant findings.

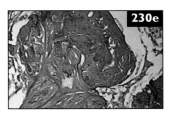

Because of the lizard's advanced age, the owner elected to have his pet euthanized and requested a full necropsy to ascertain the cause of his animal's lameness and apparent pain. Figure 230d shows the bilateral carpal foci in the upper half of one femur, and several enlarged digits.

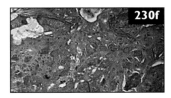

While trying to cut sections from the bony growths, it was discovered that the bone comprising these excrescences was so flinty that only after several days of decalcification in formic and dilute nitric acids was it possible to incise them. H&E-stained histological sections of the bony growths are shown in Figures 230e–g. Note the mosaic pattern of cement lines in all of these three images.

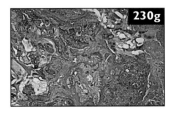

i. From this information, what are some provisional diagnoses that would be consistent with this animal's clinical signs and postmortem examination findings?

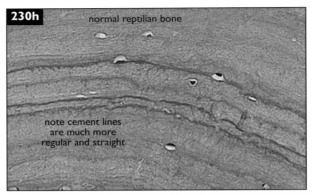

230 i. Osteitis deformans (Paget's disease of bone).

COMMENT: the author has observed this interesting condition in numerous snakes, especially boa constrictors and several crotalid pit vipers; this was the first and only case that he has seen in a reptile other than a snake.

NOTE: normal reptilian bone is characterized by its regular cement lines. For comparison purposes, see Figure 230h.

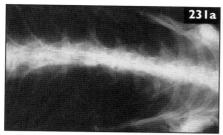

231a Dorso-ventral radiograph of iguana's thorax.

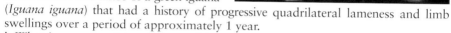

231 Figures **231a**, **231b** are radiographs of the thorax and limbs of a green iguana (*Iguana iguana*) that had a history of progressive quadrilateral lameness and limb swellings over a period of approximately 1 year.

i. What is your provisional diagnosis?

ii. What tests or procedures would you employ to confirm your diagnosis?

iii. What are some etiologies for this condition?

A whole blood specimen was submitted for a full panel. The most relevant results are provided in the table below:

Date	Test	Result	Normal values
11-3	SGOT	213 IU/l	200–300 IU/l
	Glucose	133 mg/dl (7.4 mmol/l)	<155 mg/dl (8.6 mmol/l))
	Calcium	9.7 mg/dl (2.4 mmol/l)	11.5–13.8 mg/dl (2.9–3.5 mmol/l)
	Phosphorus	ND	5.8– 6.7 mg/dl (1.9–2.2 mmol/l)
	Total protein	4.0 mg/dl (40 mg/l)	4.5 mg/dl (45 mg/l)
	Uric acid	8.1 mg/dl (0.5 mmol/l)	<5.0 mg/dl (0.3 mmol/l)
11-13	SGOT	253 IU/l	200–300 IU/l
	Glucose	ND	<155 mg/dl (8.6 mmol/l)
	Calcium	ND	11.5–13.8 mg/dl (2.9–3.5 mmol/l)
	Phosphorus	ND	5.8–6.7 mg/dl (1.9–2.2 mmol/l)
	Total protein	2.8 mg/dl (28 mg/l)	4.5 mg/dl (45 mg/l)
	Uric acid	6.8 mg/dl (0.4 mmol/l)	<5.0 mg/dl (0.3 mmol/l)

231 i. The first provisional diagnostic possibility is a metabolism-related bone disease, HPOA, which should be ruled out first.

ii. Diagnostic radiography revealed only mild apical pulmonary infiltrative changes, but significant periosteal proliferation involving all of the appendicular long bones.

When the owner was informed of the radiographic findings, she requested that her iguana be euthanized and gave permission for a necropsy. One of the forelimbs was defleshed, a small piece was cut with a hacksaw, and the balance of the limb was cleared in potassium hydroxide before it was photographed (**231c**). Cutting the bone with a new hacksaw blade was difficult because the bone was so flinty. Note the thickened compact bone radiating outward from the humeral bone marrow cavity and the enlarged radius and ulna. This specimen when completely dried weighed over 49 grams. Considering the size of the iguana, the weight of this bony specimen was substantially greater than expected.

iii. Although this condition is termed hypertrophic pulmonary osteoarthropathy, any and all of the following are capable of inducing these striking bony alterations:
- Many chronic pulmonary conditions.
- Any of several neoplasms.
- Chronic parasitism involving the lungs, heart or esophagus.
- Chronic infections and non-infectious inflammations.
- Chronic hepatic conditions.
- Chronic renal conditions, especially urinary bladder diseases.
- Chronic enteropathies.
- Chronic cardiac and/or great vessel conditions.
- Aneurysms.
- Soft-tissue, especially vascular, mineralization.

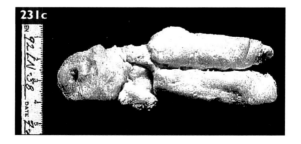

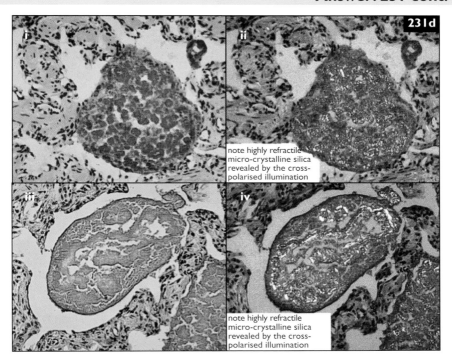

note highly refractile micro-crystalline silica revealed by the cross-polarised illumination

note highly refractile micro-crystalline silica revealed by the cross-polarised illumination

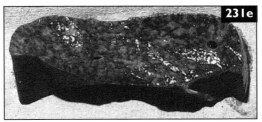

231d Paired plain illumination (i, iii) and cross-polarized micrographs (ii, iv) of pulmonary exudate. Note the refractile crystalline material revealed by the polarized illumination.

Further investigation disclosed that the crystals were from diatomaceous earth-derived cat litter to which the iguana was exposed.

231e Gross appearance of 'nutmeg' liver from the iguana.

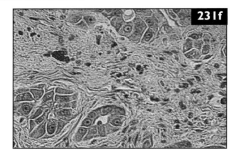 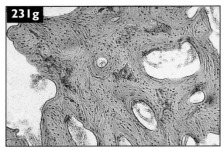

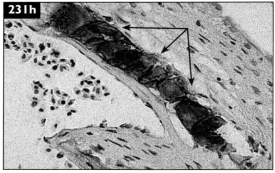

231f Histological section of the fibrotic liver. Note the widely distributed bands of fibrocollagenous connective tissue that separate islands of hepatocellular tissue.

231g Photomicrograph of a section of acid-decalcified long bone. Note the very dense compact bone and the large population of osteocytes, and the almost total lack of bone marrow elements.

231h Photomicrograph of a stained histological section of myocardium in which a portion just below the endocardium had undergone soft tissue dystrophic mineralization (arrows). This alteration was scattered throughout the myocardium

Thus, this iguana's HPOA could have been induced by any of several pathological lesions. However, it is most likely that the etiology for this disease process in this animal was the disseminated distribution of the glass-like mineral crystals in its lungs.

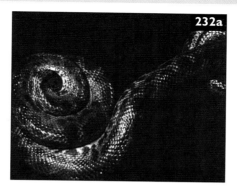

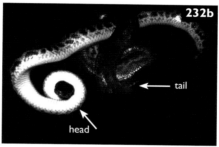

232 In Figures **232a**, **232b** an adult Children's python (*Antaresia childreni*) is displaying an abnormal posture. The cranial portion of the body and a short length of the caudal portion are tightly coiled, with the middle of the snake flaccid or partially atonic.
i. What is your tentative diagnosis?
ii. What tests or procedures would you employ to confirm your diagnosis?
iii. If your tentative diagnosis is correct, what is your prognosis?
iv. What advice would you give to the owner of this snake?

132 i. The snake is exhibiting severe neurological abnormalities and is unable to move in a co-ordinated manner. These signs can be attributable to any of the etiologies listed below:

- A meningoencephalitis due to a bacterial, fungal organism, viral agent, protozoan or metazoan parasitic infestation.
- A traumatic injury to the brain.
- An intoxication from an environmental substance, such as a pesticide, toxic gas, cleaning agent, etc.
- A metabolic dysfunction, leading to an abnormal accumulation or deficiency of an essential metabolite.
- A nutritional deficiency of an essential vitamin or ionic mineral necessary for normal neurological function.
- A space-occupying lesion such as a neoplasm or cyst or aneurysm.

ii. Useful laboratory analytical tests are a complete blood count, an analysis of physiological processes, such as blood glucose, uric acid, calcium, phosphorus, potassium, globulin, albumen, cerebrospinal fluid, etc. Once any abnormality is identified further testing is directed toward that dysfunction. In this case, there was evidence of chronic infection. The white blood count revealed a leukocytosis as follows:

Heterophils	31%	Monocytes	17%*
Lymphocytes	31%	Basophils	3%
Azurophils	18%	Eosinophils	0%

A significant number of monocytes contained engulfed bacteria. Based upon these findings, the owner elected to have his snake euthanized and requested a thorough necropsy. Figures **232c, 232d** illustrate the most significant gross pathological lesions. Note the multifocal raised gray-pink lesion on the parietal surface of the lung (black arrows).

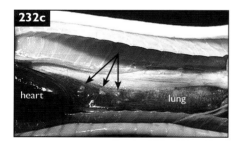

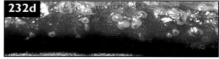

A granulomatous lesion was also found in the nasal cavity while examining thin sections of the decalcified skull of this snake (**232e**, arrow). Histology showed acid-fast microorganisms (**232f**, **232g**, Fite's stain). The confirmed diagnosis was mycobacteriosis with multifocal pulmonary and cephalic granulomata. The species of the *Mycobacterium* was not characterized.

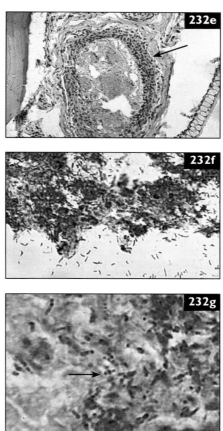

Appendix (English and Latin names)

alligator, American	*Alligator mississippiensis*
axolotl	*Ambystoma* sp.
caiman	*Caiman crocodilus*
chameleon	
East African	*Chamaeleo dilepsis* (and others)
Fischer's	*Bradypodion fischeri*
Jackson's	*Chamaeleo jacksoni*
Meller's	*Chamaeleo melleri*
panther	*Furcifer pardalis*
veiled	*Chamaeleo calyptratus*
crocodile, American	*Crocodyus acutus*
frog	
bullfrog, African	*Tromptema (Pyxicephalus) adspersus*
bullfrog, American	*Rana catesbiana*
clawed, African	*Xenopus laevis*
horned, Argentine	*Ceratophrys ornata*
leopard	*Rana pipiens*
tree	
North American	*Pseudachris (Hyla)* sp.
red-eyed	*Agalychnis callidryas*
White's	*Litoria caerulea*
iguana	
Fiji	*Brachylophus faciatus*
green	*Iguana iguana*
ground/rhinoceros	*Cyclura cornuta*
rock (West Indian)	*Cyclura nubila* sp.
spiny-tailed	*Ctenosaura* sp.
lizard	
agama	*Agama* sp.
alligator	*Elgaria* sp.
anole, Carolina	*Anolis carolinensis*
beaded, Mexican	*Heloderma horridum*
collared	*Crotaphytus collaris*
dragon	
water, Asian	*Physignathus concincinus*
bearded, Australasian	*Pogona vitticeps*,
Rankin's	*Pogona henrylawsoni*
fence ('swift')	*Sceloporus occidentalis*
fringed	*Chlamydosaurus* sp.
gecko	*Acanthodactylus* sp., *Coleonyx* sp., *Eublepharis* sp., *Gekko* sp., *Gonatodes* sp., *Hemidactylus* sp., *Nephrurus laevis*, *Phelsuma* sp., *Phytodactylus* sp., *Shaerodactylus* sp., *Tarentola* sp.

leaf-toed	*Phytodactylus* sp.
leopard	*Eublepharis macularius*
Tokay	*Gekko gecko*
Gila monster	*Heloderma suspectum*
'glass snake'	*Ophiosaurus ventralis, Anniella pulcra*
horned	*Phrynosoma* sp.
molloch	*Moloch horridus*
monitor	
mangrove	*Varanus indicus*
Nile	*Varanus niloticus*
savannah	*Varanus exanthematicus*
water	*Varanus salvator*
night	*Xantusia vigilis*
skink	
blue-tongue	*Tiliqua gigas*
New World	*Eumeces*, sp., *Scincella* sp., *Scincus*, sp., *Lerista* sp.
Old World	*Chalcides* sp, *Corucia* sp., *Egernia* sp., *Mabuya* sp., *Tiliqua* sp., *Trachydosaurus*, sp.
prehensile-tail, Solomon Island	*Corucia zebrata*
tegu	*Tupinambis teguixin (T. nigropunctatus), T. rufescens*
uromastyx, ornate	*Uromastyx ornata*
salamander	*Ambystoma* sp.
snake	
anaconda	*Eunestes marinus, E. notaeus*
boa	
constrictor	*Boa c. constrictor, Boa constrictor imperator*
rainbow	*Epicrates* sp.
rosy	*Lichanura trivirgata*
tree, emerald	*Coralus caninus*
tree, Malagasy	*Sanhzinia madagascarensis, Boa mandrita*
bull	*Pituophis melanoleucus sayi*
cobra, spitting	*Naja nigricollis*
copperhead	*Agkistrodon contortrix*
corn	*Elaphe guttata*
cotton mouth water moccasin	*Agkistrodon piscivorus*
garter	*Thamnophis s. sirtalis*
gopher, California	*Pituophis catenifer*
hog-nosed	*Heterodon platyrhinos, H. nasicus, Lioheterodon adigascarensis*
indigo	*Drymarchon corais*
king	*Lampropeltis getulus* sp.
banded, North American	*Lampropeltis alterna*

snake *(continued)*

California	*Lampropeltis getulus californiae*
gray-banded	*Lampropeltis mexicana alterna*
marine (sea)	*Acaltptophis peroni, Aipysurus duboisi, Astrotia stokesii, Emydocephalus annulatus, Hydrophis sp., Lapemis hardwicki, Laticauda sp., Pelamis sp.*
milk, Mexican	*Lampropeltis triangulum*
pine	*Pituophis melanoleucus*

python

blood python	*Python curtus*
Burmese	*Python molurus bivittatus*
dwarf, Central American	*Loxocemus bicolor*
Children's	*Antaresia childreni*
reticulated	*Python reticulatus*
rhinoceros	*Cyclura nubula*
rock, Indian	*Python molurus*
royal (regal)	*Python regius*
racer, blue, North American	*Coluber constrictor*
rat	*Elaphe sp.*

red-tailed, Asian	*Gonysoma oxycephala*
Trans-Pecos	*Bogertophis (Elaphe) subocularis*
rattlesnake, diamondback	*Crotalus sp. (C. atrox)*
taipan, Australian	*Oxyuranuis scutellatus*
vine	*Oxybelis aeneus*

viper

European	*Vipera berus*
Gaboon	*Bitis gabonica*
rhinoceros	*Bitis nasicornis*
Russell's	*Vipera russelli*
water	*Nerodia (Natrix) cyclopion, Enhydris sp.*
worm	*Rhamphotyphlops barmina*
terrapin, diamondback	*Malaclemys terrapin*

toad

marine	*Rhinella (bufo) marina*
spade-foot	*Scaphiopus sp.*
Surinam	*Pipa pipa*
western	*Bufo boreas*

tortoise

Chilean	*Geochelone chilensis*
desert	*Xerobates (Gopherus) agassizi*
Greek	*Testudo graeca*
gopher	*Gopherus polyphemus*
Hermann's, European	*Testudo hermanni*
leopard, African	*Geochelone pardalis*

pancake, East African	*Malacochersus torniei*
red-legged	*Geochelone carbonaria*
spurred	*Geochelone sulcata*
star, Indian	*Testudo elegans*
Texas	*Xerobates (Gopherus) berlandieri*
yellow-footed	*Geochelone denticulatus*
turtle	
alligator snapping	*Macrochelys temminckii*
Blandings	*Clemmys blandingi*
box	*Terapene carolina*
box, Asian	*Cuora amboinensis*
green sea	*Chelonia mydas*
hawksbill marine	*Eremochelys imbricata*
loggerhead sea	*Carretta carretta*
map turtle	*Graptemys geographica*
mata mata	*Chelys fimbriata*
mud	*Kinosternon* sp.
musk	*Sternotherus* sp.
painted, Western	*Chrysemys picta belli*
pond, Pacific	*Arctremys marmorata*
Reeve's	*Chinemys reevesi*
side-necked, African	*Pelusios* sp. (e.g. *P. williamsi*), *Chelodina expansa*
slider, red-eared turtle	*Trachemys scripta elegans*
soft-shelled turtle	*Apalone* sp.
snake-necked turtles	*Chelodina* sp., *Hydromedusa* sp.
snapping turtle	*Chelydra serpentine*

NOTE: names in parentheses were previous taxonomical classifications that have been superseded by newer names.

Index

Index

Index